A Vital Force

A Vital Force

Women in American Homeopathy

ANNE TAYLOR KIRSCHMANN

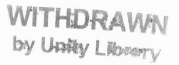
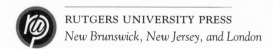
RUTGERS UNIVERSITY PRESS
New Brunswick, New Jersey, and London

3|07

Library of Congress Cataloging-in-Publication Data
Kirschmann, Anne Taylor, 1944–
A vital force : women in American homeopathy / Anne Taylor Kirschmann.
xiii, 230 p.   cm.
Includes bibliographical references and index.
ISBN 0-8135-3319-8 (hardcover : alk. paper) — ISBN 0-8135-3320-1 (pbk. : alk.
paper)
1. Homeopathic physicians—United States—History.   2. Homeopathy—United
States—History.   3. Women physicians—United States—History.   4. Women in
medicine—United States—History.   I. Title.
RX51.K55 2003 2004
615.5'32'082—dc21   2003005990

British Cataloging-in-Publication information is available from the British Library.

The publication program of Rutgers University Press is supported by the Board of
Governors of Rutgers, The State University of New Jersey.

Manufactured in the United States of America

For Peter

Contents

Preface and Acknowledgments

Several years ago at the beginning stages of my research on the history of homeopathy, I had the pleasure of spending several days perusing Edward Atwater's extensive library of American popular medicine. Atwater, a Rochester, New York, physician and educator, has since donated this exceptional collection to the Edward G. Miner Library at the University of Rochester; but at that time, it filled every nook and cranny of his home library. During my first visit, I mentioned that my grandfather, Gardiner Pratt Taylor, had graduated from Hahnemann Medical College in Philadelphia in 1904. I knew, of course, that Hahnemann had been a homeopathic college, but I assumed that by the time my grandfather attended, it had become a "regular" institution. Consulting an alumni directory, Atwater located not only Gardiner Pratt Taylor but also my great-grandfather William Gardiner Taylor, an 1860 graduate. The knowledge that my great-grandfather had also earned his medical degree at Hahnemann, and that both he and his son had been homeopathic physicians came as a complete surprise to me. No one in my family ever referred to them as homeopaths, and like many other homeopaths in the early decades of the twentieth century, my grandfather had blended into the mainstream medical landscape—known simply as "Doc Taylor" to his devoted patients and many friends.

A few years later, well into my research on this book, I received a list of names of ancestors from my cousin Gardiner Snyder who was tracing the family genealogy. Several names lacked biographical information, including two that held particular interest for me: Richard and William Gardiner. At this stage in my research, I was quite familiar with all things homeopathic, and I recognized that Richard (1793–1877) and his son William were among the original organizers in 1848 of the Homoeopathic Medical College of Pennsylvania—the first homeopathic medical college in the country and the precursor to Hahnemann University. William Gardiner was professor of anatomy at the college, and his brother, Daniel, was in the school's first graduating class.

The Gardiners were pioneers of the "new school" of medicine and prominent members of Philadelphia's homeopathic community. With this information, it became clear to me that among those to whom I owe a debt of gratitude for their guidance and help in making this book possible, I must first acknowledge these ancestral spirits. Others who have aided in the book's development have been no less inspiring but, indeed, more corporeal.

This work originated as a doctoral dissertation at the University of Rochester. I am especially grateful to Theodore M. Brown and Lynne Gordon who read multiple drafts of chapters and offered invaluable criticism and encouragement. It was my great good fortune to have had the opportunity to study with such gifted scholars. Naomi Rogers, whose work on women in sectarian medicine first gave me the idea for this project, has been an enthusiastic and constructive mentor over the years. John Haller Jr., Regina Morantz Sanchez, and Nancy Hewitt provided valuable critiques of the manuscript, and I thank them for the generous use of their time and expertise. This project benefited greatly from the expert editorial and production assistance of Audra Wolfe and Marilyn Campbell at Rutgers University Press, and from the very skillful copyediting of Nancy Condry. I extend a heartfelt thank you to Philip Ayers and Ellen Idler for their work in creating such a beautiful cover photograph.

This book would not have been possible without the cooperation and assistance from the staffs of various libraries and historical societies, including the Historical Society of Pennsylvania; Ohio Historical Society; Miami County Historical Society; Academy of the New Church Swedenborgiana Library; Arthur M. and Elizabeth Schlesinger Library; Cleveland Health Sciences Library; New York Academy of Medicine Library; Francis A. Countway Library of Medicine; Alumni Medical Library, Boston University School of Medicine; Edward G. Miner Library; Syracuse University Archives; Dittrick Museum of Medical History Archives; and the National Center for Homeopathy. I extend my appreciation to William Kirtsos for allowing me to work with materials in his extensive private collection of homeopathic books and journals and to Richard Moskowitz for his loan of several rare books during the course of my research. I owe a special debt of gratitude to Barbara Williams of the Archives and Special Collections on Women in Medicine and Homeopathy, Drexel University College of Medicine. Barbara's indefatigable interest in the history of homeopathy and her dedication to preserving its past enabled me to work with materials that most likely would have been relegated to the very real dustbin of history. Barbara's knowledge of the homeopathic collection, her indispensable assistance, and her enthusiasm and support, contributed mightily to this project.

I take great pleasure in thanking several institutions for the financial support that helped make this work possible. Early stages of my dissertation research were supported by a University of Rochester Rush Rhees Fellowship for Graduate Interdisciplinary Study. During the summer of 1994, I spent several weeks at the Medical College of Pennsylvania (now part of Drexel University College of Medicine), as a recipient of the M. Louise Carpenter Gloeckner, M.D., Summer Research Fellowship. F. Michael Angelo, Director of Archives and Special Collections on Women in Medicine, and Teresa R. Taylor, Associate Archivist, provided valuable assistance and made my stay there a most pleasant one. The following summer, I was the recipient of a Resident Research Fellowship at the Francis Clark Wood Institute for the History of Medicine, College of Physicians of Philadelphia. Thomas Horrocks, Director of Historical Programs and Services, and Monique Bourque, Assistant Director for Programs, made available to me the vast resources of the Institute's collection. Historical Reference Librarian, Charles Greifenstein, made sure "my cart" was constantly replenished with requested books and journals and facilitated a gazillion photocopy requests. For their hospitality, good humor, and valuable assistance, I thank them.

Julian Winston, Librarian and Archivist for the National Center for Homeopathy, deserves special mention for without him, a significant portion of this book could not have been written. During the time he was preparing to move to New Zealand, Julian agreed to meet with me to discuss homeopathy's more recent history. I was invited to his home, a converted fire station in the Kensington area of North Philadelphia, where the enormous ground-floor bays were brimming with everything homeopathic—books, journals, files, bottles, and remedies, to name a few. Picking our way among stacks of boxes, Julian invited me to "have a look." When I discovered that several boxes contained historical records of the American Foundation for Homoeopathy, I realized I could expand my work on women in homeopathy (especially lay women) beyond the nineteenth century. I was elated, but at the same time disheartened, knowing that within a few months this extraordinary collection of documents could be on its way to New Zealand. When I asked Julian if he intended to take the materials with him, he said he would rather not—that he would like to give them to someone for safekeeping, but had not yet decided who that would be. I managed to convince him that I would be an excellent choice. I appreciated their importance and would use them to expand knowledge of homeopathy's history. Afterward, I would deliver them to any location he named for permanent safekeeping (hopefully a major archive where they would be cataloged and made available to other scholars). After some discussion, he accepted my offer. We loaded the boxes into my car, utilizing every square inch of space; and I left Philadelphia that day with primary sources that would keep me busy for another four years. Besides the loan of these important materials, Julian has been an invaluable source of information and support throughout my years working on this project, and I extend to him my deep appreciation.

Many people currently active in the homeopathic community have given most generously of their time in helping me to understand homeopathy's resurgence in the late twentieth century. Physicians, physicians' assistants, nurse practitioners, and lay advocates alike discussed with me their introduction to homeopathy and their experiences as homeopathic practitioners. Most particularly, I would like to thank Katherine Vargo, Lauren Fox, Richard Moskowitz, Lia Bello, George Guess, David Wember, Lisa Harvey, Allen Neiswander, Nicholas Nossaman, Karl Robinson, Joseph Lillard, and the late Maesimund Panos and Henry Williams.

Portions of Chapters four and seven have been published previously and are used here with permission: "Adding Women to the Ranks, 1860–1890: A New View with a Homeopathic Lens," *Bulletin of the History of Medicine* 73 (Fall 1999): 429–446: and "Struggle for Survival: The American Foundation for Homeopathy and the Preservation of Homoeopathy in the United States, 1920–1930," Martin Dinges, ed., *Patients in the History of Homoeopathy* (Sheffield, UK: European Association for the History of Medicine and Health Publications, 2002): 373–387.

Lastly, I wish to acknowledge my family and friends for their steadfast support and encouragement over the years of this project. I am grateful everyday that I am the daughter of Margaret Alton Taylor and William Gardiner Taylor, who convinced me I could do anything. My own children, Michael, Ingrid, and Dana have been among my biggest fans. The title of head cheerleader, however, goes to my husband, Peter. Besides remedying countless computer glitches, he has spent hours organizing, printing, and proofreading this manuscript. During our many years together, he has been a source of unconditional love and encouragement. I am overwhelmed by his generosity.

As the reader will note, two forms of the word "homeopathy" are used throughout the book. I have retained the older, European version of homoeopathy as it appeared in direct quotations as well as in titles of early homoeopathic publications, organizations, and institutions. In all other instances, I have used the Americanized "homeopathy," which became popular in the last decades of the twentieth century.

Abbreviations

AFH	American Foundation for Homoeopathy
AIH	American Institute of Homoeopathy
AMA	American Medical Association
BU	Boston University
CPP	College of Physicians of Philadelphia
HMCC	Hahnemann Medical College of Chicago
IHA	International Hahnemannian Association
NAWSA	National American Woman Suffrage Association
NCH	National Center for Homeopathy
NWSA	National Woman Suffrage Association
NYMCHW	New York Medical College and Hospital for Women
WEIU	Women's Educational and Industrial Union
WMCP	Woman's Medical College of Pennsylvania

A Vital Force

Introduction Homeopathy as "Other"

AS ONE OF TROY, Ohio's, most prominent citizens, Mary Belle Brown's death on July 13, 1924, was front-page news. Articles recounted Brown's forty-year career as a distinguished New York physician, surgeon, and educator. They described her former residence—a brownstone mansion located off Fifth Avenue, where the names of her neighbors and some patients included Carnegie, Vanderbilt, Huntington, and Rockefeller. After a long and successful career, Brown returned to Troy in 1917, remaining active in the Red Cross during her retirement. Local obituaries noted proudly that "New York papers" also recognized the significant accomplishments of one of Miami County's most respected and successful citizens.[1] However, the otherwise informative, memorials left out the one detail of Brown's career that initially drew me to her. Rather than a member of the "regular" medical profession—to use the terminology of the day—Brown was a homeopath. She graduated from a woman's homeopathic medical school and was active in homeopathic professional organizations and institutions throughout her life. Brown's choice of homeopathy—as a profession and as a system of healing—was what intrigued me most.

Within the last few decades, scholars have provided a more complete picture of the history of women in the medical profession.[2] Recent work on sectarian medicine has revealed the significant role of women in the growth of "unorthodox" medical systems and therapeutics in the nineteenth century, including the hydropathic or water-cure movement, eclectic medicine, osteopathy, and the healing methods of Christian Scientists and Seventh-Day Adventists.[3] Yet, despite the considerable numbers of women who entered the homeopathic profession, nothing within the existing scholarship enabled me

to understand Mary Belle Brown's choice of homeopathy—the medical system presenting the most significant institutional and economic challenge to
"regular" medicine in the nineteenth century. Prior to beginning research on
this book, I viewed women such as Mary Belle Brown as the "medical other"—
women in a male-dominated profession whose affiliation with an "irregular"
medical system further marginalized them. As part of a medical system the
orthodox medical community considered marginal at best and heresy at worst,
they appeared to struggle, not only as the "other" because of their sex, but also
as the "other" medically. My thinking was influenced by the disparaging language used by both homeopaths and "regulars" (conventional physicians) in
the nineteenth century when referring to each other—terms still in use today.

Regular physicians referred to homeopaths as "irregulars," members of a
medical "sect,"—implying an anti-intellectual devotion to a medical creed
akin to religious fundamentalism. And according to homeopaths, "so-called
regular physicians" belonged to an outdated "old school" of medicine. They
named them "allopaths," a derisive term implying a lack of scientific principles or logical basis for therapeutics.[4] But what did it mean to be part of what
regular physicians called a medical "sect"? What were the motivations and
experiences of patients and physicians who chose homeopathic over orthodox
therapeutics? Were there professional and personal advantages, rather than
simply disadvantages to women who became homeopaths? As these questions
drove my research, I came to realize that the legacy of accusatory rhetoric contributed to a distorted view of medical history in the nineteenth century,
exaggerating the differences and obscuring the similarities—both professional
and therapeutic—between regulars and homeopaths. By these lights, women
homeopaths, indeed all homeopaths, were considered outside the bounds of
medical professionalism, a view that was contrary to what emerged as I explored
the professional lives of women homeopaths, as well as female patients and lay
practitioners who chose homeopathic medicine.

As John Harley Warner has shown, the homeopathic critique of heroic
therapeutics played a significant role in the decline of debilitating depletive
therapies before the Civil War and stimulated the development of an orthodox ideology by regular physicians. Medical therapeutics was the pivot upon
which the orthodox/sectarian conflict turned in the antebellum period.
Absent other means of defining professional identity and esteem such as formal education, licensing, or medical society membership, therapeutic practices were the most conspicuous symbols of homeopathic and regular identity.
Both medical groups dramatized and exaggerated their respective differences in
ideology and therapeutic practices. The trope of "otherness" used by homeopaths and regulars during that period to depict homeopathy had a long-lasting

legacy, especially among historians who, for the most part, still view homeopaths as eccentric sectarians whose medical system began and remains beyond the professional pale.[5]

By the late 1860s, however, when significant numbers of women entered the profession, homeopathic physicians increasingly used distinctive remedies in conjunction with practices and procedures commonly employed by regular physicians. The study of homeopathic therapeutics in women's diseases reveals that the presumption of homeopathic difference influenced some patients' choice of individual homeopathic physicians as well as their expectations of treatment; and physicians sometimes tailored their practices to conform to such expectations. A major challenge for homeopaths in the last third of the nineteenth century was to maintain distinctiveness, yet simultaneously advance along the path of medical progress.

While the claim to therapeutic distinctiveness remained the hallmark of difference between homeopaths and regulars, formal medical education, membership in medical societies, and the reinstitution of licensing in the last third of the nineteenth century increasingly defined "legitimacy" for both sorts of physicians, decreasing the importance of therapeutics and blurring the boundaries between the two professions. Historians' concentration on the disparaging language of physicians and the "rules" of conduct regulating regular physicians' behavior with those outside the profession has obscured the realities of practice. For example, in 1879, with the rhetoric of difference at its highest pitch, Boston homeopath Mary Safford Blake enjoyed cordial professional relationships with male regular physicians. With a general practice consisting of men, women, and children, Blake was asked to consult with a "well-known old school male physician" in one of the neighboring towns. "He sends me many patients to examine . . . [and] . . . I have operated once for him while he assisted."[6] Homeopath Sophia Penfield of Danbury, Connecticut, said she was treated with "respect" by "old school practitioners . . . willing to render me any assistance in the way of a consultation that can be held between the two schools."[7] Many similar examples confirm that in everyday practice, the lines between female homeopaths and male regular physicians were not as tightly drawn as we have assumed. However, despite the fact that women homeopaths and regulars often belonged to the same social and civic organizations, until late in the nineteenth century the professional lines between them were more rigid.

The struggle by women for acceptance into the regular medical profession was intimately bound to issues of sectarianism and the construction of orthodoxy. Regular male colleagues believed women unusually credulous and susceptible when it came to medical sectarianism, and debates on women's admission to regular medical societies reflected the view that women were more prone to this type of intellectual "instability."[8] Thus, demonstration of orthodoxy was of special concern to women regulars for whom professional intercourse with women homeopaths carried greater risks than for male colleagues. Yet, re-examining the concept of the "other" through women's professional roles in homeopathy reveals the many social, cultural, and professional similarities women homeopaths shared with women in the regular profession.

Alike in race, class, and economic background, both groups tended toward general, obstetric, and gynecological practice where women were the majority of patients. They were equally interested in preventive medicine and criticized excesses in gynecological surgery. The influence of social structures and cultural mores on health and disease of women were largely the concern of women physicians—homeopathic or regular. And both groups were influenced in their choice of career by family tradition and/or personal experience with illness. However, women's choice of homeopathy as a profession was influenced by additional factors, including expectations and assumptions of therapeutic difference as well as homeopathy's links with social reform movements, especially women's rights. In addition, the homeopathic profession provided, not only a route to a medical career, but also liberal opportunities for women to integrate and influence the direction of homeopathic organizations and institutions. While separatism characterized the careers of women regular physicians throughout the nineteenth century and beyond, an impressive level of inclusion defined those of women homeopaths, enhancing homeopathy's appeal and strengthening its identity as a progressive, forward-looking alternative to the male-dominated culture of the regular profession.

After the turn of the twentieth century when educational reforms raised admission standards, lengthening and increasing the cost of a medical education, the numbers of women in both professions declined. By this time, the professional barriers between the two groups had softened, and distinctions between homeopathic and orthodox therapeutics became less important through the transforming ideals of a universalized medical science. Leaders in both professions believed knowledge derived from laboratory experimentation, rather than theory, dogma, or professional rules of ethics, would direct clinical practice and identify legitimate physicians.

By the early 1920s, most homeopathic medical schools had closed or repudiated their association with homeopathic medicine, and homeopathic practitioners followed various routes to assimilation in the medical mainstream. Although intraprofessional relations were at their lowest ebb, women attempted to bring a state of cohesion to the profession, sustaining homeo-pathic identity and practice. But changes in patients' expectations as well as physicians' desires to conform to the standards of mainstream medical profes-sionalism influenced the ways homeopaths responded to their appeals. Inter-views of patients and physicians conducted by social reformer Mary Ware Dennett, special representative to the American Foundation for Homoeopa-thy (AFH) in the 1920s, shed light on why homeopathy declined, in what form it survived, and why some patients continued to support it. Reports of Dennett's interviews are instrumental in revealing important changes in the meaning of homeopathy, feminism, and professionalism by 1930.

Although the profession declined considerably during the middle decades of the twentieth century, homeopathy today has benefited from a resurgence of interest beginning in the late 1960s when feminists and others of the sixties generation sought alternatives to mainstream medicine. Today approximately 167 independent study groups in thirty-eight states have affiliated with the National Center for Homeopathy (NCH), in which interested lay people learn to use homeopathy for self-limiting conditions such as colds, coughs, and flus, as well as chronic illness.[9] For many, homeopathy's appeal is based, not only on its holistic approach to healing and its easily procured, gentle remedies, but also the knowledge that it is not simply "another passing fad."[10] Homeopathy's intellectual complexity, sense of tradition, and two-hundred-year-old history lend it legitimacy. And similar to the spread of homeopathy in the nineteenth century, women and the ideals of feminism have spurred its latest resurgence.

Today, as in the past, homeopathy exists within a strong female culture. Mothers are most likely to seek homeopathic physicians and practitioners for their own and their children's health problems.[11] Women constitute the majority in independent-study groups and are often group leaders, mentoring those interested in becoming professional homeopathic practitioners. Ac-cording to the 1998 *Directory of the National Center for Homeopathy*, women comprise approximately 40 percent of health care practitioners in the United States whose practices are devoted wholly or in part to homeopathy.[12]

The meaning of women's choice of homeopathy changed over time, but it was never just about medicine. Linked to social reform movements in the nineteenth century, antimodernism in the late nineteenth and early twenti-eth centuries, and to the countercultural ideals of the 1960s and 1970s, women's advocacy of homeopathy was and is intertwined with broad social and cultural issues in American society. While part of the history of science, the history of women in homeopathy contributes new understandings of feminism, women's strategies of professionalization, patients' influence on medical practice, and the changing meanings of science in medicine.

The stately home in which Mary Belle Brown was born and raised still stands about a mile outside the center of Troy. It rests amidst acres of fields once cultivated by the Brown family. Now windowless and in need of repair, its huge columns list precariously on the slowly sinking veranda. The formerly magnificent Greek Revival mansion, once such a fitting symbol of the town's most distinguished homeopathic physician stands, at least for now, as a poignant reminder of a more prosperous past.

Chapter 1

The New School of Medicine, 1820s to 1880s

Homeopathy, a medical system developed by the German physician Samuel Hahnemann in the late 1700s, made steady gains geographically, economically, and institutionally throughout the nineteenth century in the United States. Introduced in the 1820s by German-speaking immigrant physicians, homeopathy attracted advocates among patients and physicians throughout the country, but especially in the urban areas of New York, Pennsylvania, Massachusetts, Ohio, and Illinois. Enthusiastic converts to the profession established medical schools, medical societies, asylums, dispensaries, and hospitals, which published popular and professional texts introducing and explaining the new system to patients and physicians.[1]

In 1860, homeopaths were 3 or 4 percent of the 55,000 physicians in the United States.[2] By the 1890s, homeopaths numbered over nine thousand, were 8 percent of all medical practitioners, and counted among their patients some of the most elite and affluent families.[3] Women figured prominently in the rapid growth of the new school of medicine. Children's dislike of nauseating and disagreeable doses of drugs prescribed by regular physicians contrasted with their positive reactions to the small, pleasant tasting doses of homeopathic remedies, which provided an "entering wedge" for the system.[4] Mothers' enthusiasm spurred the acceptance of homeopathy as families and entire communities embraced its benign therapeutics.

As homeopathy's popularity grew, it became an important route to a medical career for women. Between 1852 and 1900, around 1,690 women graduated from homeopathic medical colleges. During the last two decades of the nineteenth century, they were 15 percent of all homeopathic medical school graduates and assumed active roles in homeopathic institutions and organizations.[5]

And laywomen, who had played an important role in homeopathy's popularity and growth in the nineteenth century, became partners with physicians to
preserve homeopathy in the twentieth century.

Of the various competing medical systems popular during the early part of
the nineteenth century, homeopathy posed the clearest institutional and economic threat to the regular medical profession. Although alternative systems
such as Thomsonism, eclecticism, and hydropathy were important means to
self-doctoring and/or a career as a practitioner, homeopathy, like regular medicine, originated within the learned European medical tradition. Although
they differed in their methods, both groups employed drugs in treating disease.
Both valued formal medical education and knowledge and developed parallel
institutional structures. And unlike anti-professional alternatives such as
Thomsonism, homeopaths were interested in and aware of developments in
medical science.

Although the term "scientific medicine" usually applies to the period
after 1870 when German laboratory medicine influenced the thinking of many
leading physicians, doctors before that time did not consider their systems of
healing unscientific. Throughout history, proponents of various medical systems claimed their methods of cure rested solidly on scientific principles, with
the definition of science and its meaning to patients and physicians in specific
places changing over time.[6] What then comprised homeopathic science, and
how did it differ from the science of the regular school? How did physicians
and patients understand the changing definition of homeopathy—what
meaning did it have for them? And to what extent did changing ideas of science influence opportunities for women in the homeopathic profession?

Beginnings

When homeopathy arrived on the American scene, the country's medical
marketplace was among the most varied in the industrializing Western world.
People relied on local midwives, granny midwives in slave communities, lay
healers, mental healers, and "Indian Doctors" skilled in the use of herbs, roots,
and other plants. Domestic medical manuals guided middle- and upper-class
patients in ministering to themselves and family members. Popular health
crusades such as those led by William Andrus Alcott (1798–1859) and
Sylvester Graham (1794–1851) promoted dietary and hygenic principles,
encouraging individuals to learn the structure and function of the body.
Botanical movements such as that led by Samuel Thomson (1769–1843),
who urged "Every Man His Own Physician," originated as a self-help movement, disdaining formal medical knowledge and training. Botanical practi-

tioners of the physio-medical sect sought to compete with regular practitioners by becoming physicians themselves, while eclectics or reformers established formal institutions for education and training beginning in the 1830s.
Through hygenic living, proper diet, and the use of cold water (internally and
externally), hydropathy, or the water-cure movement, held out the promise of
individual perfectibility, and by extension, the perfectibility of society as a
whole.[7] By the middle of the nineteenth century, spurred by the antiauthoritarian, egalitarian ethos of Jacksonian democracy, regular physicians' claims
to exclusive, arcane medical knowledge were challenged by a myriad of health
reformers and sectarian practitioners who attacked, not only the debilitating
therapeutics of physicians, but also the exclusivity of medical knowledge.

Within mainstream medicine during the early decades of the nineteenth
century, practitioners were primarily unschooled and became doctors by
apprenticing themselves to practicing physicians. A small number attended
medical schools in the United States. Fewer still studied at elite medical
schools in Europe. No licensing system required demonstration of the principles and practice of medicine. And although they were an important means of
continuing education for practitioners in rural areas or small towns, medical
journals and medical societies were not yet the instruments of professional
association they later became.

Early nineteenth-century theories of disease and maintenance of health
emerged primarily from European centers of medical education. The Hippocratic doctrine of humoralism had eroded, replaced by mechanistic views of
illness. Iatromathematicians held that the human body functioned by quan-
tifiable numbers, weights, and measures. The eminent Dutch physician Herman Boerhaave (1668–1738) posited a hydraulic model of the body, viewing
disease as an imbalance of internal fluid pressures. The work of Giovanni Bat-
tista Morgagni (1682–1771) in Italy fueled interest in pathological anatomy,
correlating symptoms with localized lesions in specific organs found on
autopsy. Others like Georg Ernst Stahl (1659–1734) from the famous Prussian
medical school, Halle, subscribed to various theories of vitalism in which an
unseen, nonmaterial *anima* or soul guided the body's physiological functions.
All assumed diet, hygiene, climate, local atmospheric states, and hereditarian
influences affected various general states of fevers, fluxes, and inflammations.
But the disease framework developed by the eminent Scottish physician and
educator William Cullen (1710–1790) had special influence throughout the
English-speaking world, shaping the practices of most American physicians by
the early nineteenth century.[8]

Cullen, chair of the Institutes of Medicine at Edinburgh in 1766, integrated earlier theories of Herman Boerhaave (1668–1738), with those of

Friedrich Hoffmann (1660–1742), and Albrecht von Haller (1708–1777), who emphasized physico-mechanical principles and the centrality of the nerves, respectively. Rejecting humoralism, Cullen theorized that all pathology originated in a disordered action of the nervous system caused by such external influences as climate, food, and humidity, and that those same factors produced different diseases in individuals. Although he agreed autopsy findings were "one of the best means of improving us in the distinction of diseases," he made little use of anatomical pathology in his own system of disease classification, a nosology categorizing an extraordinary number of different diseases according to the state of the "nerves" and clinical signs or symptoms—a system similar to those developed for plants by naturalists.[9]

Two of Cullen's pupils were particularly relevant to American medicine. Scottish physician John Brown (1735–1788) and American Benjamin Rush (1746–1813) typified the excesses of systematists who claimed their theories were based solidly on natural law. According to Brown, disease was caused either by an excess or deficiency of nervous "excitability,"—the body's capacity to react to external stimuli. Too much reaction resulted in *sthenic* diseases, requiring depletive techniques such as bloodletting, emetics, and cathartics. Too little produced *asthenic* conditions requiring the administration of opium, alcohol, and other stimulants. Brunonian medicine found willing converts in German-speaking Europe and Italy, while in the United States Benjamin Rush combined Brown's system with theories of hematological excitability, recommending massive bloodletting and other depletive therapies such as calomel—a purgative compounded of mercury.[10]

For Cullen, the treatment of disease—the correction of imbalances—was a delicate art requiring the proper timing, sequence, and dosage of medicines. But for Brown, Rush, and their followers, bloodletting to the point of unconsciousness and large doses of noxious drugs were the treatments of choice, which initiated the "heroic" age of medicine, and, in turn, stimulated the rise of alternative medical systems opposed to harsh therapeutics. In the United States, eclecticism, hydropathy, homeopathy, and the botanical systems of Thomsonism and physio-medicalism enjoyed wide popularity by the middle of the century. But unlike the populist orientation and origins of other movements, homeopathy had been developed by a German scholar and physician trained in the learned European medical tradition, reflecting the mainstream medicine of his day.[11] His new school of medicine appeared as a rational alternative to the debilitating, depletive, and stimulating therapeutics in use by regulars and attracted a number of American physicians and patients from select circles to the rival profession.

Samuel Christian Frederick Hahnemann (1755–1843) received a doctor of medicine degree in 1779 from the University of Erlangen. Although enrolled as a medical student at the University of Leipzig in May 1775, in 1777 he transferred to Vienna, where the clinical aspects of medical training were based on the model developed at Leiden by Gerhard van Swieten (1700–1772), a disciple of Hermann Boerhaave. A gifted scholar, Hahnemann had mastered nine languages by the age of twenty-four and had financed his medical education by giving language lessons to fellow students and translating French and English texts on medical and chemical subjects. After graduating, and for the next thirty years, Hahnemann restlessly moved from place to place throughout the German-speaking areas of Europe, practicing medicine for short periods of time in various locations. Growing disdainful of the common practices of bloodletting, phlebotomy, and the use of drug mixtures as emetics and purgatives, he turned full-time to writing, translating scientific texts, and the study of botany, pharmacology, and especially chemistry.[12]

In 1790, while translating William Cullen's *A Treatise on the Materia Medica* into German, Hahnemann became intrigued by Cullen's explanation for the tonic or strengthening effect of cinchona (Jesuit's bark) to treat fever, and sought to substantiate Cullen's theory by conducting experiments upon himself. For several days, he took four drams of "good china" twice daily, noting that the symptoms associated with intermittent fever appeared in succession (but in milder form). After two to three hours, symptoms disappeared, recurring when he repeated the dose.[13] Hahnemann spent the next six years noting the effects of ever-smaller doses of different drugs and poisons on healthy persons, publicizing his findings through medical lectures. In 1796 he published "New Principle for Ascertaining the Curative Powers of Drugs," outlining for the first time the law of similars (*similia similibus curantur*, or "let likes be treated by likes").[14] In 1805 Hahnemann produced a collection of drug tests or "provings," *Fragmenta de Viribus*. In 1810, the *Organon of Rational Healing* described homeopathy's laws, principles of therapeutics, and methods of proving and manufacturing drugs. Referring to the dominant school of medicine and practice as "old school," "allopathy," and "old medicine," Hahnemann intended not merely to reform medicine, but to revolutionize it.[15]

For Hahnemann, disease consisted of the totality of its symptoms, changes in the health of the body and mind "observed by the physician" and "felt by patients." It resulted from a disturbed "spirit-like" vital force—an immaterial "being" animating the material organism, manifesting disease in sensations and functions or "morbid symptoms."[16] At times, Hahnemann referred to the vital force as a physiological principle; at other times, a spiritual energy.[17] From his drug experiments, he concluded that the curative power of medicines depended on their "symptom similarity" to diseases.

Symptoms could not be alleviated by a specific drug unless the substance had produced symptoms similar to those of the disease when tested on healthy persons. Testing (proving) a drug on the healthy, and recording the reactions of provers revealed a drug's particular "characteristic." The physician's task was to choose a single drug whose characteristics most closely matched a patient's disease symptoms—one "homeopathic" to them. He theorized that a similar, artificial disease produced by the drug substituted itself for the "natural" (original) disease, causing it to disappear, reflecting common knowledge that one disease drove out another. Because of the minuteness of the medicinal dose, the artificial disease would soon be extinguished by the vital force, "striving to return to the normal state."[18]

Although Hahnemann did not claim discovery of the law of similars, he believed his drug experiments demonstrated and confirmed the practices and views of others, citing the common use of small amounts of parsley juice to promote urination; opium to treat constipation; and belladonna to cure hydrophobia—all known to cause similar symptoms when given in large doses. He pointed to the use of heat-producing oil of turpentine or alcoholic spirits to remedy burns, promoted by Thomas Sydenham and other respected medical theorists.[19]

In 1811, Hahnemann published the first volume of *Materia Medica Pura*, a compilation of his drug provings, listing medicines and symptoms caused by each. He emphasized the importance of continually proving drugs, adding to the homeopathic materia medica, and expanding upon those already tested. Homeopaths were proud of their materia medica, stressed its historical development and methodology, and considered the work of determining the pathogenesis of drugs an essential part of their role as physicians in perfecting a "vital element" of their science.[20] Several decades later in an effort to upgrade the materia medica, homeopaths in the United States called for more comprehensive drug testing on women. According to homeopathic theories of drug pathogenesis, men's and women's responses to the same drugs differed in part because of sexual difference. Therefore, in order to treat women's illnesses more effectively, they were enlisted in the important work of drug testing. Knowledge of women's early inclusion in testing homeopathic drugs was part of homeopathy's appeal to late-twentieth-century feminists critical of women's exclusion from formal drug trials in the United States.

The second major component of Hahnemann's system was the use of infinitesimal doses of drugs. Because Hahnemann viewed the essential cause of disease as invisible rather than material—caused by disorder or imbalance in the body's vital force—it was not the material, medicinal properties of drugs that restored health, but their spirit-like essence or "conceptual medicinal energy." The vital force responded to the "dynamic energy" present only in the smallest or "minimum dose," which contained so little material substance that its "minuteness cannot be thought and conceived by the best arithmetical mind."[21]

The complicated process of dynamization, or increasing a drug's potency, involved frequent triturating or mixing with potable alcohol or milk sugar upon every dilution, and many succussions or shakings. This mechanical procedure, according to Hahnemann, changed the crude drug, eliminating it altogether from the remedy, developing its "true, inner medicinal essence." The higher a drug's potency, that is, the more dilutions it was subjected to, the more powerful it was. He insisted only a single remedy be given to a patient at any one time, with the "gentlest and most rapid cure" depending not only on its accurate selection but also on its proper dose. He urged physicians to determine the most suitable degree of minuteness on careful observation of the sensitivity of each patient. Homeopathy's emphasis on the individual was another part of its appeal to late-twentieth-century critics who viewed mainstream medicine as the epitome of a depersonalized and dehumanized bureaucratic system.

Like several other vitalist medical theorists in the eighteenth century, Hahnemann defined disease as the totality of an individual's symptoms. He ridiculed the attempts of "old school" physicians to discover the essential nature of disease, believing it unnecessary to know how a deranged vital force produced symptoms. The only imperative was to remove them, thus extirpating the entire internal and external morbid state. He rejected the naming of diseases, saying it led to medicinal conformity, whereby treatment was based on the single most prominent symptom associated with the disease rather than the individual's unique physiological reaction to it. Acknowledging the necessity of using names when talking to "ordinary persons," Hahnemann suggested physicians use terms such as "a *kind* of dropsy" or "a *kind* of typhus."[22]

In 1828, Hahnemann completed the first of three volumes of *Chronic Diseases, Their Individual Character and Homoeopathic Treatment*, explaining his theory of psora. Added to later editions of the *Organon*, the theory was rejected by many adherents, leading to decades of controversy.[23] Chronic diseases, said Hahnemann, stemmed from inherited "miasms" such as syphilis or sycosis (wart-like skin eruptions), including the miasm of "psora"—the "fundamental cause" underlying all. Of long-standing duration, characterized by skin eruptions reflecting the internal diseased state, psora produced a multitude of symptoms experienced by those diagnosed with hysteria, mania, epilepsy, gout, cancer, impotence, barrenness, and other conditions. Treating external psoric manifestations locally, without employing "anti-psoric" internal homeopathic remedies to treat the hidden infection, was not only useless, but positively harmful, driving the miasm deeper into the body and making it most difficult to treat. Along with the dimunition of remedies to a point where no material part of the original drug remained, the doctrine of psora became a source of conflict among American homeopaths almost from the beginning.[24]

Homeopathy's roots in the United States were established in New York and Pennsylvania. Boston-born Hans Burch Gram (1786–1840), the son of Danish immigrants, graduated from the Royal Medical and Surgical Institute in Copenhagen where he developed an interest in homeopathy. Returning to America in 1825, Gram began practicing homeopathy in New York City, attracting converts to the new system which gradually spread among both patients and physicians throughout New York, New Jersey, and New England. In the 1830s, numerous German immigrant communities in Pennsylvania supported the efforts of William Wesselhoeft (1794–1858), Constantine Hering (1800–1880), and Henry Detwiller (1795–1887) to establish the first homeopathic medical school in Allentown, Pennsylvania—the North American Academy of the Homeopathic Healing Art or Allentown Academy. Hering, later dubbed the "Father of American Homeopathy," founded several homeopathic medical schools and societies, and wrote over forty books and pamphlets, including the most widely used materia medica (*Condensed Materia Medica*) and home health manual (*The Homoeopathic Domestic Physician*).[25] In the 1840s, practitioners carried homeopathy into the Midwest, some going as far as California. Many of these practitioners were natives of Germany or of German extraction. Some had been pupils of Hahnemann, and others were graduates of the Allentown Academy where instruction was entirely in German. By the middle of the nineteenth century, homeopathy was established in sixteen states, and had attracted the attention of many urban middle-class families and intellectuals.[26]

As Naomi Rogers argues, homeopathy is best understood as a form of "complementary medicine" during this early period. Practitioners only gradually came to view themselves as "fully antagonistic" to orthodox medicine, committed to revolutionizing rather than improving it.[27] Many were regular physicians who had converted to homeopathy, but remained members of orthodox medical societies. During this period, homeopaths and regulars held common views on the predisposing causes of disease and the physician's role in curing it.

Both groups believed that most debility and disease resulted from destabilizing factors or exciting causes such as cold, anxiety, or improper behavior relating to food, drink, fresh air, sexual activity, and exercise, rather than specific causative agents. The physician's objective was to restore the patient to a natural state of health, using therapies based on an individual's symptoms, the physician's knowledge of a patient's personal and family history, individuating factors such as gender, ethnicity, moral status, constitution, and temperament; and an assessment of contributing factors including region, locale, and climate. Homeopaths and regulars alike claimed a commitment to therapeutic specificity—individualizing therapies according to patient and place. Until its gradual erosion toward the end of the century, this model of medical holism informed patients' and physicians' understanding of disease and their respective areas of responsibility in the doctor/patient relationship in both schools of medicine.[28]

Homeopathy's benign therapeutics as well as its testing of harmless drugs on healthy persons, rather than experimenting on the ill or on animals, was a commonsense selling point to patients. Figuring prominently in literature designed for the lay audience, it represented an important difference between homeopathic and regular medicine.[29] Several scholars have noted that in their attention to precise methods of observation and exactness in accumulating data for provings, homeopaths appeared more scientific than regular physicians. As one observed, Baconian principles of inductive philosophy were so pronounced in homeopathy that ". . . the regulars' efforts to achieve orderliness and numerical precision seemed bumbling and feeble" compared with those of "homeopaths."[30]

Although conducting provings was the work of physicians, a full account of drug reactions required both male and female provers. Physicians amassed data on provers' psychogenic and physiological reactions to drugs in various areas and functions of the body including: eyes, ears, mouth, and nose; the heart, lungs, and sexual organs; elimination, breathing, sleeping; and pregnancy, among others. Because women's and men's sexual organs and function were obviously different, physicians enlisted both male and female provers in developing drug characteristics for the materia medica, an essential element of homeopathic science.

A typical proving took place over a period of weeks, during which a prover (usually a medical student or patient chosen by a physician) took drugs of specific doses and potencies at intervals directed by the doctor. Noting symptoms reported by the patient (termed subjective) and observing the patient's reactions (referred to as objective symptoms), physicians recorded almost verbatim provers' descriptions of physical sensations, thoughts, and feelings. Narratives of "symptoms" from many provers formed the basis for a drug's mental, emotional, and physical "characteristics."[31] Doctors based their choice of remedy on the similarity between a drug's characteristics and the patient's symptoms, often placing greater importance on mental and emotional symptoms than strictly physical ones. According to Hahnemann, the "condition of the disposition and mind is *always* altered" in disease, providing the more "striking, singular, uncommon, and peculiar" signs and symptoms, leading to the correct remedy.[32]

For example, a doctor whose patient experienced "tardy menstruation," would not necessarily choose a remedy based on that primary complaint, but on the presence of idiosyncratic symptoms related to the patient's disposition or temperament.[33] One physician said if he met a person with a "pure *Pulsatilla* temperament," he would almost always find that the patient's physical symptoms and conditions corresponded in kind to the drug derived from the wind-flower.[34] For particular drugs like Pulsatilla, the disposition and mental state were the chief guiding symptoms to the selection of a remedy.

While provings were essential in developing knowledge of drug action, the physician's role in "taking the case" was important for the application of this knowledge. For homeopathic science to work, patients needed to supply an accurate and full description of symptoms. Advice to physicians on the art of case taking urged doctors to develop techniques of questioning to produce a vivid, accurate account of a patient's physical, mental, and emotional states. They were directed to let the patient tell her story in her own way without interruption, recording the case "as far as is practicable" in her own words. One methodologist suggested that the physician "should follow the patient absolutely in the unfolding of the history in whatever direction it goes."[35] And in a pamphlet designed to help patients communicate with physicians through letters when a personal visit proved impossible, James Tyler Kent reminded patients their communications would be held in the strictest privacy: "No one will ever learn of your private troubles or symptoms through the agency of your physician. Therefore be perfectly free in your statements."[36]

Often patients articulated fears, anxieties, and frustrations contrary to Victorian assumptions of proper gender roles and behavior. Men wept, expressed indifference to their children, their hatred of work and friends, and confessed to irrational thinking. Women disclosed "immodest" behavior, boredom with domestic duties, and feelings of aggression toward husbands. Women as well as men may not have shared such feelings with friends or family members. As a character in Elizabeth Stuart Phelps's popular novel *The Story of Avis* (1877) pointed out, a "terrible competition" isolated women from each other. "That's the worst of being a woman. What you go through can't be told. It isn't respectable for one woman to tell another what she has to bear."[37]

Obviously shared confidences were not unique to the homeopathic patient/physician relationship. Some regular doctors knew a great deal about their patients' lives—their worries, fears, and difficulties past and present. Recent scholarship using physicians' case narratives show the extent to which this knowledge figured into the decisions southern doctors made concerning kind, amounts, and frequency of medicines.[38] But some physicians deliberately cultivated aloofness in their relationships with patients to ensure the respect they felt they deserved.[39] Others discounted the value of communications with particular groups of patients. For example, one regular physician advised a young colleague not to attach great importance to the words of upper-class patients: "With the wealthy and pampered . . . there is often such a concatenation of unrelated or chronic symptoms, or they are described in such diluted or exaggerated phrases . . ."[40] To the extent homeopaths conformed to correct case-taking procedures, the doctor/patient relationship consisted of physicians encouraging patients to elaborate upon any and all sensations or emotions, however irrelevant they seemed. Besides aiding physicians in the correct choice of remedy, the obvious therapeutic benefit of talking was psychological. But patients' emotions and thoughts—like their physical sensations— were considered part of the anatomy of illness, symptoms of a deranged vital force no different from pains in the legs or back, except for their sometimes greater importance to physicians in choosing remedies.[41]

Patients' words, even their self-absorption, were important clues leading to a physician's success. But if homeopathic patients learned no detail was too small to be of interest to conscientious doctors, the task of homeopaths, like regular physicians, was to distinguish between patients' reliable and unreliable symptom accounts. Although some may have listened longer and more patiently, homeopaths shared regular physicians' distrust of symptoms reported by some women, mostly those diagnosed with nervous disease.

Recounting his experience with a neurasthenic patient, Boston homeopath Conrad Wesselhoeft said her exaggerated introspection complicated his task considerably. For two hours, Wesselhoeft dutifully recorded her "innumerable sensations," filling several pages of his notebook. His tongue-in-cheek assessment of the patient's "keynote" symptoms, those most expressive of her illness, was: "neurasthenic patients have innumerable sensations and exhibit no signs of fatigue after talking incessantly for nearly two hours."[42]

We cannot know how many homeopaths followed the model of case taking, sometimes lasting one to three hours. For those who did, the importance of patients' cooperation and full revelations perhaps led to patients' awareness of their special, if not equal, role in healing. As one doctor said, "When things seem to be going wrong, I try to impress patients with the idea that they may be as much or more to blame than the physician."[43] While the role of patients served a utilitarian purpose for some physicians in deflecting criticism when treatment failed, homeopathy's "science of therapeutics" placed high value on patients' involvement, awareness, and articulation of their illness experience. Women's and men's emotions were not discounted as irrelevant by practitioners, but were essential clues in selecting remedies, perhaps enhancing homeopathy's appeal for members of both sexes. A century later, this aspect of homeopathic science and practice would hold special appeal for feminists challenging the superiority of doctors' so-called objective clinical knowledge over subjective knowledge based on women's own experiences of their bodies.

Growth and Development

Homeopathy underwent a period of rapid growth between 1830 and 1860, a period when leading orthodox physicians increasingly turned away from speculative systems of disease based on a new theory of empiricism learned in the great hospital clinics of Paris. As elite American physicians returned from advanced clinical instruction in Parisian clinics, they spread the ideals of a new medical science through positions as teachers, editors of journals, and authors of medical articles. They urged colleagues to reject medical theory and dogma, promoting instead knowledge based on direct observation of patients through a cultivation of the five senses and the analyses of pathological lesions found at autopsy.[44] The study of normal and pathological anatomy as well as mastery of technical and conceptual tools such as the stethoscope, scalpel, and statistical studies comparing large numbers of patients, formed the core of a new empiricism. Paris-influenced doctors stressed the careful recording of facts by observing patients' symptoms, responses to percussion, palpation and auscultation, and postmortem examinations, constructing a natural history of disease. Autopsy findings and bedside observation linked disease to anatomical pathology.[45]

Regular physicians who supported the new empiricist program believed increased knowledge of disease would hasten the decline of heroic practices, demonstrating the progressiveness of regular medicine and forming the basis for a new definition of science in medicine, elevating it in the minds of the public and the profession.[46] Disciples of the Paris School led the crusade against both orthodox and anti-orthodox speculative systems such as Brounianism, Thomsonism, hydropathy, homeopathy, and "all systems of medical delusion."[47] As John Harley Warner argues, regular leaders "sharpened the dichotomy" between orthodoxy and homeopathy by identifying the latter with a repudiated past—a "dogmatic, unprogressive, and doctrinaire" system doomed to extinction.[48] According to Warner, framing homeopathy in this way "was a powerful means for regular physicians to imagine themselves set apart from it by chasms in epistemology and integrity alike. An ideology of orthodoxy configured this way made its bid both for absolute separateness and for the moral high ground."[49]

Within the competitive atmosphere of mid-nineteenth-century medicine, homeopathy had attracted significant numbers of middle-class intellectuals, especially in urban areas of the Northeast. Its assault against heroic drugging had influenced many physicians in prescribing milder therapies. And from its identity as a populist movement earlier in the century, it had established itself as a competing profession—with medical schools, dispensaries, professional journals, and societies. Institutionally, professionally, and in its system of therapeutics and drug testing, homeopathy was distinct from other popular health reform movements and alternative medical systems. For the majority of homeopaths, their system was a superior tool in the treatment of disease, not alternative medical knowledge. They located themselves firmly in the Hippocratic tradition of healing and believed it was only a matter of time before regular physicians would see the error of their ways.

In 1844 homeopaths established the American Institute of Homoeopathy (AIH). Partly in response to homeopathy's growing popularity, regular leaders formed the American Medical Association (AMA) in 1847. One of the new organization's first official actions was the adoption of a code of ethics, including a consultation clause separating legitimate physicians (orthodox practitioners) from all others. The clause forbade professional association or consultation with physicians whose practices were based on an exclusive dogma. Anyone calling himself or herself a homeopath was considered an "unfit" associate in consultation, regardless of the wishes and needs of patients.[50] The clause was a key instrument in aggravating tensions between homeopaths and regulars; and for the next few decades, rhetoric from both sides exaggerated differences and obscured similarities in their ideologies and practices.

Although the earliest homeopathic medical schools were distinctive in their teaching of homeopathic materia medica and therapeutics, they conformed to the organizational structure and taught the standard medical topics of the day.[51] There was no special "homeopathic" understanding of obstetrics and gynecology; chemistry and toxicology; surgery, physiology, and pathology; or medical jurisprudence. And while some of the earliest educators considered themselves "pure" homeopaths, upholding Hahnemann's tenets and framing homeopathy as completely antagonistic to regular medicine, homeopaths disagreed over Hahnemann's more controversial theories such as the "doctrine of psora," dynamization, and the value of "high potency" remedies. Most viewed themselves part of a progressive school of medicine whose therapeutics and investigative techniques in drug testing would be informed by new knowledge and technology, advancing along with medical science. And, as homeopaths sought to conform to new standards of evidence stemming from Parisian empiricism, many criticized the drug provings found in homeopathic materia medicas.

Although the testing of drugs was a stated goal in founding the AIH, it offered little in terms of organizational help, oversight, economic support, or ground rules. Drug testing was usually the work of individual physicians, who often published results in books or pamphlets, and/or submitted them to a myriad of homeopathic journals. Editors compiled provings from these sources both in the United States and abroad, publishing multivolume editions of homeopathic materia medicas.[52] Beginning in the 1860s, leading homeopathic reformers questioned the reliability and quality of drug provings. In 1866, a member of the American Provers Union of the AIH spoke for many of his colleagues when he criticized the "thousands of fragmentary provings which flood our journals and which, of themselves, are of no value whatever."[53] Members attending the AIH meeting in 1874 had equally poor opinions of the reliability of physician-provings performed "without much forethought or critical care."[54] During a discussion at the World Homoeopathic Convention in 1876, participants criticized the quality of provings in the *Encyclopedia of Pure Materia Medica* edited by Timothy Field Allen. One individual argued that twenty-two drugs had gone through no form of proving, sixty-eight had but one prover each, thirty but two provers, etc., leading him to estimate that over one-third of the entire number had no methodical proving whatsoever upon the healthy or else a simple trial by one prover each. Discussions reveal criticism of unreliable data, incompetencies of "average" homeopathic physicians, and the "perversion" of homeopathic science by "high-potency" advocates.[55]

Around this time, several prominent homeopaths argued that the improvement of the materia medica necessitated women's full acceptance into the homeopathic profession. Traditionally, female provers were often "healthy" patients of doctors—women whom physicians believed would conscientiously follow their instructions on dosages and timing of remedies and report accurately on their symptoms. But most were doctors themselves or medical students, who were considered preferable to patients because of their superior intellect, education, and training. There were few women homeopathic medical students before the middle of the 1860s. Leaders pointed to the "weakness" of the materia medica for its lack of reliable information on the physiological effects of drugs upon women's "peculiar organism." They argued that women physicians possessed the requisite accuracy and intelligence to conduct provings, but would be unlikely to take part in the work unless accorded the "respect" and status of males in the profession.[56]

Ruben Ludlam, one of homeopathy's foremost gynecologists, believed women homeopathic physicians were especially important in homeopathy's ability to treat women patients suffering from nervous diseases. Patients' "incidental, irrelevant . . . and hysterical symptoms," he said, confused the careful homeopathic physician in choosing a remedy. Ludlam believed untrained women provers could not be trusted to report accurately on their symptoms, necessitating the training of "intelligent" women doctors who would be able to provide "non-hysterical, non-exaggerated information" in proving homeopathic remedies for use in treating nervous diseases.[57] Mercy B. Jackson, one of Boston's first female homeopaths, urged her "Fellow-laborers in the cause of medical science" to recognize women's special abilities to interpret the symptoms of infants, noting their "peculiar insight" into the signs of infantile suffering. Citing the precedent of Marie Melanie d'Hervilly, Hahnemann's second wife, Jackson reminded her colleagues that homeopathy's "great founder" educated his wife to be a homeopathic physician. Jackson encouraged Hahnemann's disciples to remember and follow their founder's example.

Thus, while arguments justifying women in regular medicine were often based on women's "inherent" qualities of tenderness, empathy, and nurturance, in 1869 male homeopaths advocated their admission to the AIH and other homeopathic medical societies, based on the "educated" woman's intelligence and accuracy in furthering homeopathic science.[58]

From Bedside to Laboratory

By the latter decades of the nineteenth century, most regular physicians agreed the influence of French medicine had increased knowledge about disease, but made few new contributions to therapeutics. An important goal of Paris-trained reformers was to end the excesses of the heroic practices of speculative systems. By 1860 they viewed the decline in depletive practices such as bloodletting and mineral cathartics an improvement over past practices. But unlike advances in experimental physiology, biological chemistry, microscopic pathology, anatomy, and diagnostic precision, there had been few new contributions to the therapeutic armamentarium.[59] Believing that so long as therapeutic decisions remained dependent only upon empirical clinical observation, therapeutics would lag behind these other areas, leaders in the regular profession suggested several routes to remedy therapeutic stagnation.

Some looked to environmental influences and personal behavior to foster nature's own healing power. Others advocated state-supported preventive medical programs. Many Paris-trained physicians favored a revitalized version of empirical clinical observation—a "rational empiricism"—as they called it, while younger colleagues trained in German laboratories and clinics looked to experimental science as the wave of the future. Proponents saw a way to ele-vate medicine through universalized knowledge derived from scientific exper-imentation. They argued that neither statistical observational knowledge nor physiological knowledge could determine the effectiveness of therapies or guide therapeutic change. Only when the bedside decisions of physicians were based on "certainties," knowledge derived from physiological laboratory experimentation, would a level of scientific accuracy be attained in prescrib-ing drugs and explaining disease. By combining clinical observation of drug action on patients with knowledge gained from laboratory experiments on animals (vivisection), advocates foresaw a way out of the therapeutic quagmire.[60]

The gradual shift from empiricism toward a new medical ethos had pro-found consequences for homeopathy. While the majority of regular physicians remained ambivalent toward laboratory science, doubting its relevance to practical therapeutics, the curricula of medical institutions and the profes-sional identities of physicians were transformed over the next several decades. Whereas a physician's identity and authority traditionally derived from adher-ence to professional ethics regulating behavior with sectarians, patients, and other practitioners, professional legitimacy depended more and more upon doctors' identification with new scientific ideals. The growing reliance on and belief in laboratory findings stimulated changes in physicians' thinking regarding sectarian medical systems. Those embracing the ideal of experimen-tal science came to believe that rules governing consultation with home-opaths and other "irregulars" were unnecessary; ideally, practices of legitimate physicians would be directed by scientific knowledge based on concrete facts, rather than dogma or theories. In several medical societies during the 1870s and 1880s, physicians debated the rationale for prohibiting consultation with homeopaths. At a meeting in February 1882, a committee appointed by the Medical Society of the State of New York to study the AMA code recom-mended a "new code," eliminating the prohibition against consultation with "any legally qualified practitioners of medicine."[61] Although the proposal failed to find favor with many other state medical societies or with the AMA (which refused to seat New York's delegates at the national meeting), the society's actions reopened the question of what constituted legitimate medical practice.

As regular physicians discussed and debated the changing standards of medical science and who should be considered a legitimate physician in light of these changes, homeopaths engaged in similar debates. Although the rhet-oric between homeopathic traditionalists and reformers seemed narrowly focused on drug potency, the issue was highly symbolic, reflecting broader professional concerns. Beginning in the 1870s, many leading homeopaths also studied in Germany, seeking specialist clinical training alongside orthodox physicians.[62] Homeopathic schools incorporated the new sciences of microscopical pathology and bacteriology into their curricula. However, the stirrings of toleration by regulars and the convergence of homeopathy with new medical ideals threatened traditionalists within the profession. Calling themselves "Hahnemannians," this group claimed to adhere strictly to the teachings of Samuel Hahnemann, viewing homeopathy as a separate medical system whose principles were wholly incompatible with regular medicine. When the AMA ostracized anyone calling themselves a homeopath from regular medical societies and prohibited consultations, homeopathic identity was fashioned as the outcast "other," no matter how lax individuals might have been in adhering to Hahnemann's basic principles. With the decline of homeopathic distinctiveness, Hahnemannians' professional tolerance of eclectic colleagues now gave way to vituperative criticism. As one physician noted, "In the hour of our bondage, when proscription stared us in the face, we were a band of brothers . . . but now prosperity makes us more vicious, and 'rule or ruin' seems to be more and more the fundamental idea of a professional life."[63]

In 1870, AIH president Carroll Dunham addressed members of that organization in a speech later recalled as a turning point for the profession. Dunham, who was a professor and dean of New York Homeopathic Medical College, was widely respected as an authority on the materia medica and renowned for the efficacy of the high-potency remedies he personally prepared. Addressing his colleagues, he acknowledged that many in the profession thought the Institute should establish admission qualifications. But despite his devotion to strict homeopathy, he argued forcefully against this move, reminding homeopaths of their own struggle for liberty against restrictive decrees of the regulars that interfered with investigation, observation, and free thought and expression, shutting out all knowledge that might have been gained from those who differed from them.[64]

Today, said Dunham, the AIH comprised many calling themselves homeopaths who did not accept all the homeopathic laws of practice: some mixed remedies in prescriptions, alternated and rotated them, and gave massive doses. But like regulars who maintained allegiance to the principles of heroic medicine, even as they downplayed or discontinued therapeutic practices based on those principles, Dunham argued that heterogeneous prescribing did not indicate disregard for homeopathic principles. He insisted that the doors of the organization should be open to all seeking membership, on the assumption that none would do so if they did not substantially accept the law of similars.

Like reform-minded regular physicians, Dunham argued against an exclusive creed and any restrictions relating to theory and practice.[65]

Dunham believed the AIH had an important responsibility to set an example and to instruct wayward homeopaths, envisioning a route to progress on this path of liberty:

> If some neophyte, fresh from the instructions of the old school, give us, in exchange for our therapeutic knowledge, some glimpses of the progress of pathology which shall show us that one day our sciences, now at variance, may be harmonized again, I think that the great object of the Institute, 'the promotion of medical science,' will thereby be more truly advanced than by any decrees of exclusion or resolution of close communion![66]

Dunham expressed the views of the majority of his colleagues, for whom liberalizing tendencies among regulars, as well as the changing ideals of science, including the clinical empiricism of the Paris School, the rise of specialties, and the more recent promotion of the experimental laboratory, evidenced progress.

In 1874 members attending the AIH meeting in Niagara Falls voted to strike the word "homoeopathy" from the requirements for membership. And in 1880, "pure" (Hahnemannian) homeopaths formally separated themselves from the majority of their colleagues by founding the International Hahnemannian Association (IHA).[67] For Hahnemannians, the greatest threat to homeopathy now lay within their own profession. Confident that developing medical knowledge would eventually support and confirm Hahnemann's principles, they feared that "poorly educated homeopaths" (those not scrupulously adhering to Hahnemann's tenets) would hide their inadequacies amidst the authoritative glow of the new medical science. Adolph Lippe, one of the most outspoken of this group and a founding member of the IHA, accused one individual claiming to represent the majority of homeopaths, of perverting the "Homoeopathic school into eclecticism, with a scientific pathologico-physiological livery exhibited, to cover the hideousness of the mongrel creature hiding under it."[68]

While physicians differed on how to incorporate the new ideals of science into homeopathy, laypersons were equally divided on the question of what constituted proper homeopathic practice. The 1887 "falling-out" between physicians and lay managers at a new homeopathic hospital in Philadelphia founded by the Women's Homoeopathic Association of Pennsylvania, showed how changing ideas of science influenced professional prerogatives, promoted alliances between physicians and lay advocates, and transcended gender and professional solidarity.

At the 1887 meeting of the IHA, members devoted considerable attention to an invited guest, Miss A. E. Ramborger of Philadelphia. A representative of the hospital and dispensary of the Women's Homeopathic Association of Pennsylvania, founded in 1884, Ramborger reported on the lay managers' work to establish a hospital in Philadelphia dedicated to homeopathy "pure and simple."[69] In their efforts to found a hospital where homeopathic principles would be carried out in their "strict integrity" by Hahnemannian standards, the women faced considerable opposition from physicians and lay supporters of Philadelphia's Hahnemann Medical College, the oldest and largest institution of its kind in Philadelphia. But Hahnemannians in Philadelphia disdained the college. They argued that its curriculum no longer reflected the teachings of Samuel Hahnemann, and instead, perverted "true" homeopathy. Philadelphia's Hahnemannians, therefore, congratulated the lay managers (all women) of the new hospital for their spirit of "bravery" and "perseverance" in establishing a hospital of the "right kind, governed by right principles."[70]

The new hospital, located at Twentieth Street and Susquehanna Avenue, was founded by seventeen Hahnemannian women who were members of the auxiliary board of the Philadelphia Homoeopathic Hospital on Cuthbert Street. As founders and fund-raisers, women concerned themselves with all aspects of the construction and operation of the new Women's Homeopathic Hospital (officially named the Medical, Surgical, and Maternity Hospitals of the Women's Homoeopathic Association of Pennsylvania).[71] Unlike most hospitals, where men assumed administrative responsibility after women raised funds and gathered support, the Philadelphia women elected themselves managers, which was supported by influential Hahnemannian leaders. Dr. Adolph Lippe took special interest in a number of the hospital's cases and was a frequent consultant; and James T. Kent, also on the consulting staff, inaugurated his post-graduate course of lectures at the hospital in 1890.

From the beginning, the lay managers provided professional opportunities for women, hiring ten female physicians who, with fifteen male doctors, comprised the medical and surgical staff.[72] In May 1887, public attention turned toward the hospital when disagreement between lay managers and the hospital's women physicians erupted in a series of letters to local newspapers over the resignation of eight "lady" physicians, all prominent homeopaths and active members of the Women's Homoeopathic Medical Club of Philadelphia. They were members of the AIH as well as county and state homeopathic medical societies. None belonged to the IHA.[73] As Ramborger reported the incident to members of the IHA, "The trouble we had was principally with three women physicians, who had brought drugs into the Hospital," in opposition to the rule that "No medicines, except strictly homoeopathic potentized remedies, shall be allowed for use in the dispensaries or in any department of the Hospital."[74] When lay managers chastised the offending physicians, eight women physicians protested—first by striking, and then by formally resigning. Two others left their positions around the same time for unknown reasons, and the annual report of 1887 lists Jennie Medley as the only remaining female physician of those originally hired.[75]

The two groups representing Philadelphia's divided homeopathic community responded through their respective medical journals. *Hahnemannian Monthly*, which no longer represented the views of "pure" homeopaths, was an organ of Hahnemann Medical College. Its articles supported the women physicians for their conscientious refusal to submit to the less knowledgeable laywomen, whose lack of medical education and training rendered them unfit to make medical decisions.[76] Critics denounced the managers for their incomplete and narrow definition of homeopathy focused on infinitesimalism or potentized remedies alone, rather than homeopathy "in its completeness." Such "delusion," one wrote, seriously harmed the cause of homeopathy.[77] Reactions of the Hahnemann College community to the resigning women physicians were driven, not only by ideological differences, but also by professional issues. They considered most homeopathic hospitals in Philadelphia mediocre, therefore compromising financial support for worthier homeopathic institutions and tarnishing the image of homeopathy. They believed physicians, not laypersons, should control such institutions. In siding with the resigning women doctors, Hahnemann College faculty upheld what they believed were the prerogatives of trained physicians to direct practices in medical institutions rather than laypersons.[78]

Hahnemannians were not surprised by the school's support of the resigning physicians, calling Hahnemann Medical College nothing but a "burlesque," having been taken over by eclectic homeopaths. By their lights, the lady managers had simply exercised their duty and were "fully competent to determine what is homoeopathic treatment and what is not . . . the managers of the Women's Homoeopathic Association know what Homoeopathy means."[79]

For lay managers of the women's homeopathic hospital, commitment to homeopathic principles and therapeutics according to Hahnemannian guidelines transcended their original support of women physicians. And perhaps more importantly, the lay managers' power and authority was upheld and strengthened by respected Hahnemannian leaders in Philadelphia at a time when hospital management was rapidly becoming the work of paid male administrators and physicians.[80] On only one point did the factions agree: the differences between them were much broader in scope than disagreement on specific drugs or the question of potency. Hahnemannians, fearing the loss of homeopathic identity, held onto what was clearly distinctive in homeopathy.

As Warner argues, therapeutic principles held symbolic function. Although bloodletting declined in practice by 1860, regular physicians continued to claim its value, in principle, to the orthodox armamentarium.[81] Heroic therapeutic principles helped to define regulars against competing Thomsonians, eclectics, hydropaths, and homeopaths, just as homeopathic therapeutic principles distinguished that system from others. In their desire to preserve homeopathic distinctiveness, Hahnemannians placed ideology above professional concerns, allying with laypeople considered competent in determining proper homeopathic practices. And although gender was a strikingly prominent element in this incident, it was subsumed by the more critical issues of changing definitions of homeopathic science and professionalism.

As this incident demonstrated, the majority of homeopaths in Philadelphia—those supporting the college's position—believed doctors alone were qualified to make medical decisions, based on their access to the latest scientific knowledge. They defined homeopathy broadly, rejecting what they called an outdated allegiance to therapeutic practices established long before the advent of new scientific knowledge. The broader issues illuminated in the debate rested on the ways homeopaths sought to redefine homeopathy in a changing medical world. And the situation in Philadelphia reflected professional trends throughout the broader homeopathic community.

Reformers argued against any special homeopathic understanding of pathology, physiology, or chemistry, insisting that the fundamental branches of medicine were the same for both schools.[82] For most, homeopathy was no longer a distinct medical system but simply a useful therapeutic specialty. Like their male colleagues, the majority of women homeopathic physicians followed the progressive route. Few women joined the International Hahnemannian Association in its early years during the 1880s. But for reasons examined more fully in later chapters, their numbers increased beginning in the 1890s.

By 1910, women Hahnemannian physicians comprised around 25 percent of the IHA—more than the percentage of women in the AIH (12 percent) and in the profession as a whole (16 percent).[83] Similar to the Philadelphia Hahnemannians, traditionalists were more interested in maintaining homeopathic distinctiveness than in professional solidarity, aligning themselves with like-minded adherents, even if they were laypersons and women. The Hahnemannian model of lay/physician cooperation became an important strategy in the twentieth century as a new generation of conservative homeopaths sought to revive an older, more spiritual, homeopathic tradition. Women were prominent among them, as physicians and lay advocates alike struggled to preserve homeopathy as a distinctive medical alternative despite the widening authority and power of early-twentieth-century mainstream medicine.

	Women Physicians,
	Lay Healers, and the
Chapter 2	Choice of Homeopathy

WOMAN'S RIGHTS LEADER Elizabeth Cady Stanton first heard about homeopathy in the 1830s through the illness of her brother-in-law, Edward Bayard. When Bayard was diagnosed with heart disease and given a bleak prognosis by a regular New York City heart specialist, Stanton's sister Tryphena urged him to consult a homeopath. Family members considered Bayard's recovery under the care of homeopath Augustas P. Biegler remarkable, and the experience so stimulated Bayard's interest in homeopathic medicine that he gave up the practice of law to become a physician. Subsequently, both Stanton and Tryphena became enthusiastic converts to homeopathy.[1]

A popular homeopathic lay healer within her community of Seneca Falls, New York, Elizabeth Cady Stanton doctored family, friends, and neighbors armed with a homeopathic domestic medical kit—one of the most important and effective tools in the propagation of homeopathy. Irish families who had settled in the area to build the Erie Canal consulted her on a variety of medical problems. Stanton was proud of her self-reliance, successfully managing her own parturitions, and of nursing her children through malaria, whooping cough, mumps, and broken limbs.[2] After the 1852 birth of her daughter, Stanton wrote to her friend Lucretia Mott describing the "easy" fifteen-minute labor and delivery of her healthy baby and rapid recovery: "Dear me, how much cruel bondage of mind and suffering of body poor woman will escape when she takes the liberty of being her own physician of both body and soul!" Stanton denounced both the Protestant and "medical ministries" for their manipulation of women, arguing that the "genteel" and "civilized" woman was made ill and unnecessarily dependent upon their authority.[3] For Stanton and other reformers, the rejection of patriarchal, unfeeling religion went hand in hand with antiauthoritarian sentiments toward established medical practices.

Elizabeth Cady Stanton's experience with homeopathy touches on several important themes linking homeopathy with various antebellum reform impulses. While homeopathy's popularity was due in large part to the public's embrace of its gentle remedies, its appeal was based, not only on a set of therapeutics, but also on homeopathy's connections to reform more broadly defined. In the antebellum period, a number of homeopathic physicians supported temperance, antiracist reform, and woman's rights, contrasting and perhaps exaggerating their support of liberal causes with conservative regulars.[4] To political liberals and social progressives, homeopathy's challenge to the regular profession, and its stated intention to reform conventional therapeutics was part of the democratization of American society and culture. Homeopathy's goal of reform appealed to groups seeking to make America's social, religious, and political institutions more inclusive. As scholars have shown, the growth of antebellum unorthodox healing movements paralleled and often intersected with unconventional religious currents. Dissenters from Calvinist orthodoxy directly challenged church hierarchies and doctrinal teachings of established religious denominations, emphasizing personal experience and conscience.[5] The egalitarianism emerging from the "age of the common man," encouraged the expression of a new kind of freedom from established authority, stressing self-reliance and the glorification of the individual. Health crusaders and social reformers, Christian perfectionists, and advocates of unconventional medicine transformed America's institutions as new themes in art, literature, and philosophy reflected the romantic movement's emphasis on intuitive knowledge and feelings—the unseen and spiritual—over the dry logic of reason. According to one historian, "many intellectuals found in homeopathy a way to link a progressive commitment to science with their faith in the primacy of spirit over matter.[6]

By the middle of the nineteenth century, prevailing cultural themes of individualism, egalitarianism, and self-reliance extended from religion and politics into the domain of health and the body. Abolitionists, woman's rights activists, Christian perfectionists, and temperance reformers shared a belief in the combined power of free will and perfectibility to effect change, stimulating antebellum interest in hygiene, physiological instruction, dietary and dress reform, as well as temperance. Good health became a personal duty, mitigating less tangible disorders in the lives of middle-class women, while enhancing their domestic authority. Seen as a key to a better society—enabling women to manage the home as well as to produce, educate, and rear healthy children—health reform included a powerful critique of established medical practices.[7] Well aware of the competitive and antagonistic relations between homeopaths and regulars, advocates used homeopathy both for practical health benefits and as a way to show disdain for more broadly defined orthodoxy. Their actions revealed a wide variety of social, religious, professional, economic, and personal factors influencing women's decisions to adopt the new school of medicine.

Homeopathy and Religious Dissent

New England transcendentalists were among homeopathy's earliest advocates. Inspired by German romanticism, believing certain truths were not susceptible to proof but transcended the limits of reason, transcendentalists valued sense perception or intuitive reason along with "pure" reason in the formation of judgments. Many were attracted to Hahnemann's metaphysical view of disease causality, his emphasis on the connection of mind and body in healing, and his insistence that only the spirit-like activity of medicinal substance (rather than the material drug) would influence a disordered spirit—the root cause of all disease.

New England transcendentalists and advocates of homeopathy included Theodore Parker, Bronson Alcott, William Lloyd Garrison, Elizabeth Peabody, and Louisa May Alcott. Peabody published a memorial upon the death of one of Boston's earliest and most distinguished homeopaths, William Wesselhoeft. A student of the Universities of Berlin and Wurzburg, Wesselhoeft earned his doctor of medicine degree from the University of Jena in 1820 before immigrating to the United States and converting to homeopathy. One of the earliest homeopaths in the United States, Wesselhoeft was cofounder of the first homeopathic medical school in Allentown, Pennsylvania, and with his brother Robert, founded the Brattleboro Water Cure in Vermont.

Peabody wrote of Wesselhoeft's "tender sensibility and disposition, love of nature," and the interest taken in his early education in Germany by Goethe, a family friend and advocate of homeopathy. Along with Wesselhoeft, Peabody was impressed with what she thought of as homeopathy's "scientific origin," Hahnemann's twenty-year experimentation and proving of drugs; yet, neither could explain (nor cared) why infinitesimal remedies worked. For Wesselhoeft as well as Peabody, positive experiences with homeopathic remedies were ultimately more important than knowledge of how homeopathy worked, allowing them to suspend disbelief in light of practical results supporting homeopathic theory. Wesselhoeft's successful treatment of patients with scarlet fever, "the terror of Boston," endeared him to many mothers and members of the city's most conservative families.[8]

Louisa May Alcott had a long-standing relationship with Boston home-opath Conrad Wesselhoeft, an 1856 graduate of Harvard Medical College and William Wesselhoeft's nephew. Alcott believed mercury, prescribed for her when she contracted typhoid fever early in the 1860s, had ruined her health and caused her chronic pain.[9] While Alcott tried a variety of cures over the years, including magnetic therapy and botanicals, she consistently relied on homeopathy and Wesselhoeft during the last twenty years of her life. Alcott's novel, *Jo's Boys* (1886), revealed the meaning of homeopathy to the author through the character of Nan. A pupil of Mrs. Jo and Professor Bhaer, Nan was portrayed as a bright, "scientifically minded" young girl who displayed her ability to remain calm in crises instigated by the Bhaers's two mischievous sons. When a dog presumed to be "mad" bit one of the boys, Nan immediately cauterized the wound with a hot poker and treated the boy with homeopathic remedies for several days. Nan was independent, smart, and dedicated to women's equality; and when she decided to become a homeopathic physician, the Bhaers encouraged her. Alcott dedicated the novel to her "friend and physician," Conrad Wesselhoeft.[10]

In addition to their advocacy of homeopathy, Alcott and other transcen-dentalists were inspired by the Swedish scientist and religious mystic Emanuel Swedenborg. Founders of the Church of the New Jerusalem, Swedenborgians were among the earliest and most consistent advocates of homeopathy throughout the nineteenth century and into the twentieth. According to one 1854 estimate, approximately 85 percent of the followers of Emanuel Sweden-borg were "enthusiastic disciples of Hahnemann." Throughout the nineteenth century, *New Church Life*, a monthly journal devoted to Swedenborgian teachings, published articles describing the "intimate relation existing between homeopathy and the Church of New Jerusalem."[11]

Although Swedenborgianism had many variations, its relationship to homeopathy rested on the similarities in Emanuel Swedenborg's and Samuel Hahnemann's teachings that disease was essentially a "dynamic alteration of the spirit." According to historian Robert Fuller, Swedenborg's concept of the deity was that of a spiritual essence flowing through all things. One had only to eliminate the barriers between the physical and spiritual planes, allowing the energy and guiding wisdom from the higher to penetrate the lower, material realm. Swedenborg's writings gave homeopathic practitioners a metaphysical rationale for infinitesimal dynamized doses of medicines. Both Swedenborg and Hahnemann postulated physical and metaphysical laws for understanding one's relationship to a "higher sphere" at a time when traditional churches and conventional medicine failed both spirit and body.[12]

Early homeopaths such as Hans B. Gram and Constantine Hering were

Swedenborgians, as were the Boericke and Tafel families, the largest and longest-standing manufacturers of homeopathic remedies throughout the nineteenth, twentieth, and into the twenty-first century. In Pennsylvania, members of the New Church were trustees of Hahnemann Medical College, and in 1890, were instrumental in founding James Tyler Kent's Post-Graduate School of Homoeopathics. With communities in Illinois, Pennsylvania, and Massachusetts, Swedenborgian women were both dedicated patients of homeopathic practitioners and physicians themselves.

Alcott's friend and confidante Rhoda Ashley Lawrence of Roxbury, Massachusetts, graduated in 1885 from the homeopathic medical school at Boston University. A Swedenborgian homeopath, Lawrence received help establishing her practice in Boston from Conrad Wesselhoeft, also a member of the New Church society. With financial help from Alcott, Lawrence founded a nursing home at Dunreath Place in Roxbury, where Louisa May Alcott spent the last years of her life.[13] Swedenborgian Mary Florence Taft, cousin of President William Howard Taft, graduated in 1886 from the homeopathic college at Boston University, where she worked closely with fellow church member William P. Wesselhoeft. After practicing medicine for several years in Waterbury, Connecticut, Taft became professor of gynecology at Hering College in Chicago, eventually returning to Boston where she practiced until retirement.[14] Homeopath Clara Louise Toby Kent, also a Swedenborgian, became the third wife of James Tyler Kent in 1896, although we know little about her educational background or practice.[15]

Transcendentalism and Swedenborgianism were important but radical manifestations of the flowering of nineteenth-century religious liberalism. Other, more common strands of evangelical Protestantism were perhaps more influential in providing a rationale for women's entrance into the medical profession. Proselytizing churches tended to support the idea that women were morally superior to men, perhaps unintentionally encouraging women to exercise their supposed moral superiority within the larger public arena. Some, like Quakerism, stressed the equality of all human beings, and were known for their support of women's rights. Similar to women regulars, women homeopaths often came from families affiliated with liberal religious denominations including Methodism, Unitarianism, Universalism, Presbyterianism, Quakerism, and Freewill Baptist.

Self-Reliance and the Domestic Medical Kit

Women's contributions to community welfare through the lay practice of homeopathy were aided by one of the most effective tools in the propagation of homeopathy—the home health manual and domestic remedy kit. The "box and book" were designed primarily to aid mothers in the treatment of uncomplicated and common illnesses suffered by family members. Home medical guides produced by regular physicians and advocates of various other medical systems were common by the middle of the century. Some described the home preparation and consumption of roots and herbs, while others provided details on the preparation of medicines from common household ingredients such as Indian meal or wood ashes. But unlike most home health manuals, whose recipes required laborious preparation and compounding of medicinal substances, the homeopathic manual was usually designed to accompany a kit containing small vials of ready-to-use remedies.[16] And unlike domestic manuals published by Thomsonians who disdained formal medical training and knowledge, the homeopathic kit was never intended to replace physicians, but to limit domestic practice to uncomplicated periods of illness or to provide help when no properly-trained homeopaths were available, gradually enlarging the constituency for homeopathic physicians.

The thousands of homeopathic domestic medical kits sold throughout the nineteenth century ranged in size from small pocket cases to large family chests. Constantine Hering developed the first kit in the 1830s. Costing five dollars, it included a copy of his *Domestic Physician* (1835) and a small mahogany box of medicines. To prevent indiscriminate self-dosing, Hering assigned numbers to the vials of medicines rather than labeling them with the names of drugs. For example, patients suffering with symptoms associated with measles were advised to give No. 8 at the first sign of symptoms or when measles prevailed in the neighborhood. "If a fever be high, give No. 3 . . . When the glands under or before the ears swell, give No. 15."[17] Hering's subsequent kits and most others named the infinitesimal remedies contained in individual vials, opening the door to lay practice. As one physician noted: "With a good family case and a good little materia medica, she [mother] will be equal to many an emergency in which she would entirely fail if she had to compound medicines after the old fashion way."[18]

The sales of two domestic guides and accompanying kits developed by Frederick Humphreys, a former professor at the Homoeopathic Medical College of Pennsylvania, were extraordinarily successful. By the 1890s, fifteen million copies (in five languages) had been sold—twelve million in the United States.[19] Homeopaths as well as regulars acknowledged the importance of the kits in diffusing the principles of homeopathy and winning converts, especially in the hands of women. As Dr. Ruddock, author of *The Stepping Stone to Homoeopathy and Health*, put it: providing laypersons with advice in self-treatment paid in the long run, "for there is no better proselyte-maker than a laywoman who has performed some miraculous cure with Aconite and Chamomilla."[20] While furthering the profession's goals, homeopathic domestic kits served women's needs as well, providing an effective means to expand women's role from caretaker of their family's health to that of lay practitioner within the community. Domestic kits appearing in the latter part of the century tended to be less comprehensive than those produced earlier, focusing largely on emergency care or minor illnesses.[21] Although homoepathic practitioners claimed patients had little need for detailed knowledge of treatment because of the prevalence of physicians, they also recognized that too much self-reliance on the part of patients was contrary to their pecuniary interests.

Often, a successful experience with a domestic kit influenced women's choice of medical career. As a teenager, one of Rita Dunlevy's proudest possessions was a small Boericke & Tafel remedy case given to her by her grandfather, Dr. Christian Ehrmann of Louisville, Kentucky. Dunlevy recalled the time a girlhood friend spent the night, only to be awakened early in the morning with diarrhea, a condition that had existed for months. Her friend, the daughter of a local druggist, reluctantly consented to take the sulphur remedy proffered by Dunlevy; and according to the latter, one dose cured her. Dunlevy later became a homeopathic physician, graduating from New York Medical College and Hospital for Women in 1888.[22] Like Dunlevy, women who entered the homeopathic profession or became lay practitioners were often influenced by their own or their family's experiences with illness.

Entering the Profession—Regulars and Homeopaths

While the popularity of domestic kits spurred interest in homeopathy, the demographics of women who chose careers in homeopathic medicine and their reasons for doing so are strikingly similar to those who became regular physicians. Nineteenth century women physicians were overwhelmingly white, from middle-class families who frequently supported their decision to study medicine. Prior to 1880, women medical school graduates were congregated geographically in the Northeast—although a significant minority of women homeopaths came from the Midwest due to early acceptance of women in homeopathic colleges in Cleveland (1852), Chicago (1871), Detroit (1872), Saint Louis (1875), and Ann Arbor, Michigan (1877).[23] Most attended seminaries, private preparatory academies, normal schools, or private colleges prior to entering medical schools. Both groups usually came from families whose religious denominations supported reform ideology. The choice between regular or homeopathic medical careers often rested on an individual's experience during a previous illness and/or family ties.

Fidelia Rachel Harris Reid who grew up in Chautauqua County, New York, underwent a painful operation on her neck "to relieve a disfigurement caused by a burn received in infancy." At twenty-seven years of age, she had long been interested in the study of physiology, and her three years of postoperative suffering made her determined to become a physician. In 1857 she graduated from Eclectic Medical College in Cincinnati and established a medical practice in Beaver Dam, Wisconsin. In 1860, after marrying homeopath and Unitarian clergyman, H. A. Reid, she turned to the study and practice of homeopathy, "retaining only a few eclectic formulas."[24]

Like Reid, women were sometimes encouraged by husbands to join them in their medical practices. Sarah Blakelee Chase, daughter of a Presbyterian clergyman from Richmond, Ohio, financed her education at Alfred University in Allegheny County, New York by teaching. In 1860 at age twenty-three, she married Hazard D. Chase, a student in the homeopathic medical department at the University of Michigan. When he returned from the Civil War, the couple studied homeopathy with Dr. Bosler of Dayton, Ohio; and in 1868, both enrolled in Cleveland Homoeopathic Hospital College. After graduating in 1870, the Doctors Chase established a practice together in Cleveland.[25] Other women were influenced in the direction of homeopathy by parents who encouraged daughters' professional aspirations.

In the 1860s Mary Belle Brown's father Daniel was one of the most prosperous farmers in Troy, Ohio, the owner of one thousand acres. Liberal Republicans and abolitionists, Brown's parents provided for her education at Oxford Theological Seminary run by the Associate Reformed Presbyterian Church in Monmouth, Ohio. After graduating, her mother encouraged her to study medicine with their family physician, the only homeopathic doctor in Troy. In 1876, Brown traveled east to study with Clemence Lozier and graduated from New York Medical College and Hospital for Women in 1879. Brown became an important figure in women's homeopathic education in New York. She was on the teaching faculty of her alma mater for twenty-seven years, served as dean from 1890 to 1898, and established a lucrative medical practice in the city.[26] Similarly, Harriet Judd Sartain's aunt and uncle encouraged her entrance into homeopathic medicine, both financially and emotionally. In exchange for their help, they requested Sartain to return to their town of Waterbury, Connecticut, to practice medicine for one or two years. After that time, her aunt and uncle promised to "pull up stakes" and accompany her to a "better location for her practice." They later released Sartain from this obligation because "it may do harm if there were no prospects for a successor to cultivate the ground which she has broken up. If she should stay a year, and the truly delicate have her services, they would suffer a great deal more by being obliged to go back to the old system."[27]

The presence of a homeopathic physician within one's family often influenced women in their choice of homeopathy as a medical career. For example, Clemence Lozier's mother Hannah Walker Harned was cousin to New York homeopath and educator Carroll Dunham. Both of Hannah Walker Harned's two children, William Harned and Clemence Lozier, became homeopathic physicians. When Lozier died on April 26, 1888, mourners included her niece and successor, Dr. Harriett C. Keatinge, nieces Anna Manning Comfort and Amelia A. Comfort of Syracuse, Jennie V. H. Baker and Emily L. Smith of Brooklyn, and her cousin, Charlotte H. Woolley of New York—all homeopathic physicians.[28]

As historians have shown, until the latter part of the nineteenth century, women often justified their choice of a medical career by using some variation on the theme of domesticity, broadly defining "woman's sphere" to include participation in public life. Women in both schools of medicine were actively involved in various overlapping visions of the nineteenth-century's woman's movement, claiming their superior moral refinement, sympathy, gentleness, and love in the sick room, especially fitted them for the medical profession.[29] Many believed domestic responsibilities were especially compatible with the practice of medicine both ideologically and practically. Combining marriage and children with a medical career was not uncommon in the nineteenth century. Recent studies show that between one-fifth and one-third of women physicians married—a rate that was disproportionately high when compared with all employed women.[30] Homeopath Anna Manning Comfort remembers the negative reactions of friends and relatives when she returned to her medical practice after the birth of her three sons. Although Comfort believed "motherhood was my nearest duty," she did not deem it incompatible with her medical career. To the "surprise and questioning" of friends she said: "I knew nothing of culinary art and I was educated to serve my sisterhood, which work I deemed yet vital."[31]

For women whose husbands died or were unable to work, a medical career offered the best way to support their families. Two national surveys published in 1881 reported annual average earnings of $2,907 for women doctors—an income roughly three times that of a male white-collar worker.[32] Others' goals conformed more clearly to a strand of the woman's movement associated with self-interest and based on equal rights.

According to Harriet Judd Sartain, a medical career was the culmination of her strong desire for economic "independence" and psychological parity.

She attended the first term of the American Hydropathic Institute in 1851, studying under Mary Gove Nichols; and in 1854 graduated from the Eclectic Medical Institute of Cincinnati, where she developed an interest in homeopathy. In that same year, Judd received a marriage proposal from Samuel Sartain, eldest son of famed Philadelphia engraver John Sartain. In response, Harriet wrote to him with details of her personal life to provide the wealthy and socially prominent Sartain family of Philadelphia with a fuller understanding of its prospective member. The letter clearly implied that Judd would sooner release Samuel from his commitment to marry her than give up her career. If the Sartains found her unacceptable because of family background or her profession, "their love could not increase as it should." In 1854 she wrote to Samuel: "I must be an independent woman, able to stand alone. When I can do that I can stand more efficiently as the other self, of a fine man." She warned that her profession was "annoying" at times—she would be called away frequently—but under no circumstances would she abandon it or use it as something "to fall back on," rather it was "something to increase if necessary."[33]

In some cases women unabashedly acknowledged that their primary interest in a medical career was its high status and potential for financial reward. When Frances Janney attended the homeopathic ophthalmology institute in New York, she boarded with Louise Gerrard, a professor at New York Medical College and Hospital for Women. Janney liked Gerrard, calling her a "dignified, fine looking young lady (thirty+) . . . [and] exceedingly refined."[34] Although she disapproved slightly of her new friend's "pride" and desire to "make money," Janney attributed these "faults" to Gerrard's English blood and former wealth.[35]

Given the similar influences on women choosing careers in either homeopathic or regular medicine, what distinguished the two groups? In what ways did women's experiences as homeopathic physicians differ? What was the meaning of a homeopathic identity to the first and second generation of women in medicine?

Feminism and Homeopathy

Although we need detailed case studies analyzing women physicians' participation in reform movements in particular locations, ample anecdotal evidence suggests that first generation women homeopaths were more conspicuous in expressing feminist ideals than women who sought assimilation into the regular profession. Women regulars often dissociated themselves from women too closely associated with suffrage and health reform, eschewing behavior which might be considered extremist by male colleagues.[36] However, the homeopathic profession was linked in peoples' minds (if not always in the behavior of individual homeopaths) with radical reform, especially women's equality. And both male and female homeopaths took advantage of the profession's liberal image to achieve professional, personal, and social goals.

Clemence Lozier, a pioneer in women's medical education, was a prominent figure in New York City reform circles. A health reformer who began her career as a teacher and lecturer, Lozier was one of the first women graduates of the Eclectic Medical School in Syracuse, New York, in 1853. Ten years later she founded the homeopathic New York Medical College and Hospital for Women, the most important institution for women's homeopathic education in the United States.[37] Jessica Lozier Payne recalled her grandmother's "gracious personality" and "gentle beauty," but noted her "forceful" character. She was an inspirational public speaker and commentator on world events, gaining results by persuasion.[38] Lozier's home at 361 West Thirty-fourth Street was a mecca for reform activity, filled to overflowing with documents and pamphlets protesting women's inequality under the law, as well as petitions on behalf of suffrage, antislavery, temperance, sanitary reform, improvement of conditions for American Indians, moral education, and reform of prisons and insane asylums. Lozier was a passionate abolitionist, hosting monthly Antislavery Society meetings. During the city's race riots of July 1862, she provided a safe haven for people of color fleeing mob violence and secured medicine and food for children of the Colored Orphan Asylum after the burning of that institution. Lozier was also one of the founders and secretary to the Female Guardian Society, rescuing "destitute and degraded women and children" from New York's prisons and slums. Among her personal friends were the most noted reformers of the day, including Elizabeth Cady Stanton, Susan B. Anthony, Mr. and Mrs. Gerritt Smith, Wendell Phillips, and Frederick Douglass.[39] She generously supported The Revolution, contributing both money and frequent articles and letters espousing woman's rights.[40] A familiar figure in the city, she led "public indignation" rallies to stimulate public outrage over court decisions or public behavior she considered unjust. Lozier was frequently aided in these rallies by her daughter-in-law Charlotte Denman Lozier, herself a homeopathic physician, labor activist, and leader of the Working Woman's Association in New York.

Alice Boole Campbell was among the first class to enter New York Homeopathic College and Hospital for Women, graduating in 1863. When her husband unexpectedly died shortly thereafter, Dr. Campbell moved her family to Brooklyn, where she built a very successful medical practice. Dedicated to the homeopathic profession, Campbell served on the governing board of her alma mater, was consulting physician on the staff of Woman's

Hospital of Philadelphia, and from the beginning of her career, strove to carve out a place for women in a male-dominated profession.[41] Campbell's strong character and belief in woman's rights led her to confront injustice. She publicly withdrew from the Methodist Episcopal Church because it did not allow women to be representatives to its conferences. Garnering national support, Campbell forced the General Conference of the Church in 1906 to right this injustice. Her refusal to compromise on important egalitarian principles was felt in her chosen profession.

Campbell was surprised and angered at the response to her application to the Kings County Homoeopathic Society in 1870. She said she received "as rough and cowardly handling from gentlemen living on the 'Heights' and the 'Hill,' (Brooklyn's elite neighborhoods) as that of the Bellevue boors," referring to the male medical students at Bellevue Hospital who taunted and insulted women attending lectures. At a meeting attended by a rather small percentage of the membership, Campbell's application was approved, and she was voted into the county organization. But as she recalled it, the doctors seemed surprised by what they had done. The meeting erupted into a "fierce wordy battle," ending with the vote nullified and set aside until a subsequent meeting when, in the opinion of some, a vote among a larger, more representative, number of members would surely result in her defeat. Not one to give up, Campbell attended all meetings of the society, stood up to be counted on all questions, and cast her ballots along with her new colleagues, who tried unsuccessfully to ignore her. With her physical presence denied, her ballots ceremoniously plucked from the box and left uncounted, Campbell decided to appeal to a higher authority. She took the Kings County Homoeopathic Society to court and won her case. "An appeal to the courts compelled the restoration of my rights, and I was reinstated at a special meeting called for that purpose."[42]

Although Campbell's experience was not typical of other women homeopaths—most did not bring suit against male colleagues—her story suggests they may have been less constrained than women regulars in their demand for equality. For example, Marie Zakrzewska, well-known educator and founder of New England Hospital for Women and Children, upbraided feminist Caroline Dall in 1867 for her published article demanding the admission of women to Harvard Medical School. Zakrzewska deemed it "overly aggressive" and impolitic, lacking the careful strategy necessary to win support for the cause of coeducation. Other leading women regulars agreed with her, believing women's interests would be best advanced by conforming to the highest standards of professionalism and shunning behavior and attitudes that would cast doubt upon their suitability as colleagues.[43]

Although it appears women homeopaths fought two battles—as the "other" in a male-dominated profession and as the "other" medically, the latter identity may have been an advantage to women seeking equality within their profession. Unlike women regulars, women homeopaths did not struggle to integrate themselves into a profession associating women with "irregular" or inferior medical training as a means to bar them from the profession. Although their entrance into the homeopathic profession was not without male opposition, women were among the earliest graduates of homeopathic medical schools. In defending those schools against regulars' accusations of inferiority, male homeopaths necessarily defended women, as well. Despite ideological and gender differences, homeopaths presented a united front when under attack by the regular profession. While regular physicians felt under siege by both women and homeopaths, leaders in the homeopathic profession considered women useful allies in their battle against allopaths, realizing homeopathy's links with progressive social reform—especially women's rights—was an important source of its popularity.[44] As a result, the profession tolerated or perhaps even encouraged greater activism among first- and second-generation women in the profession. Examples include Susan Edson and Caroline Brown Winslow, two of the earliest women graduates of a homeopathic medical college.

An 1854 graduate of Western Homoeopathic College in Cleveland, Ohio, Susan Edson is best remembered as personal physician to President James Garfield and his family. Edson, along with homeopath Caroline Brown (later Winslow) helped establish the National Woman Suffrage Association (NWSA) in 1869. Winslow, who graduated two years after Edson from Cleveland's homeopathic college, was elected vice president of the NWSA in 1873. Both women came to Washington, D.C., during the Civil War to nurse wounded soldiers and remained afterward to form the nucleus of an active female homeopathic community centering around the Homoeopathic Free Dispensary. Along with the dispensary established by women homeopaths and lay supporters, in 1873 Winslow founded the Moral Education Society, whose broad agenda promoted suffrage, voluntary parenthood, divorce, temperance, dress reform, and provided financial aid to striking women workers. Almost every woman homeopath in the city belonged to one or both of these organizations. Late in the 1880s, Caroline Winslow also played a leading role in organizing the District Woman Suffrage Association, (called Wimodaughsis, an acronym for wives, mothers, daughters, sisters), which was primarily concerned with establishing national headquarters for NWSA in Washington, D.C., and a local chapter of the Women's Educational and Industrial Union (WEIU).[45]

The WEIU was originally organized in 1877 by Boston homeopath Harriet Clisby, an 1865 graduate of New York Medical College and Hospital for Women. Promoting the ideology and politics of sisterhood, the organization challenged both class and gender inequalities by actively recruiting women from Boston's diverse constituencies—from the elite of Beacon Hill and Back Bay to the large immigrant population (estimated to be one-third of the city in 1880) crowded into the North, West, and South Ends.[46] Now, over a century later, the WEIU is still located on Boylston Street in the heart of Boston.

Unlike a labor union, the WEIU brought together the "family" of women. Founders hoped women could be first convinced of their own value and then become interested in the needs of others of their sex, regardless of differences in class, race, religion, ethnicity, or perceived morality. Clisby believed goals of economic and intellectual self-reliance for all women fostered by "bonds of love and mutual service" would shatter indifference and mistrust, fostering true sisterhood. By the end of the first year, the organization grew from eight to four hundred members. In 1887, its membership was twelve hundred, and a plethora of services aided women's educational, industrial, and social advancement, including: training and job placement for the handicapped (often defined as women "handicapped" by race or age); vocational training; lunchrooms for working women; evening classes; a handicraft workshop and sales room; health education, including free medical treatment; employment services for college women as well as domestic servants; milk distribution; and legal aid for needy women.[47]

The founding of the WEIU expressed one of the major intellectual themes of the woman's movement in the nineteenth century—its critique of inequities inherent in industrial capitalism organized on the basis of individualism and competition. Similar to earlier utopian socialist visions and utopian communities, the WEIU attempted to create awareness of how America's economic system promoted race, class, and gender conflict rather than cooperation. As historian Nancy F. Cott points out, the communitarian socialist tradition was a resource for women who sought public acknowledgment and discussion of important issues such as the sexual division of labor and the relation of the private household to the rest of society.[48]

In addition to Clisby, the first board of directors included Arvilla B. Haynes and Mercy B. Jackson, both prominent Boston homeopaths. Many early and long-lived members of the organization, including Julia Ward Howe, Edna Dow Cheney, Abby May, Abby Diaz, and Mary Livermore, had close ties to transcendentalists, had been active in the abolitionist movement, or lived at Brook Farm. Organizers sought diversity on their board of directors, which included Mrs. Louis Brandeis, African American reformer Josephine Ruffin, and Irish Catholic labor organizer Mary Kenney O'Sullivan.[49] Women physicians were directors of "hygiene and physical culture" as well as "moral and spiritual development." From 1877 to 1887, all WEIU physicians were homeopaths.

Mary Safford (later Blake) was one of the WEIU's first physicians. An 1869 graduate of New York Medical College and Hospital for Women, Safford traveled widely in Europe, engaging in clinical work at General Hospital in Vienna and the University of Breslau in Poland, where she performed surgeries and studied microscopy and obstetrics under Breslau's leading specialists.[50] After locating in Boston, Safford was appointed chair of diseases of women at Boston University's homeopathic medical college and became well-known for her reform activities. Her students, however, did not always approve of her advanced opinions. Frances Janney complained about her professor's radical attire and ideas, including her promotion of free love. Janney assured her mother, who was a "social progressive," that she herself remained neutral. However, her letters suggest that in the milieu of the college and perhaps in Boston itself, Janney's opinion was in the minority and she was reluctant to be identified with the anti-progressive "other side."[51]

As Janney noted, one of Mary Safford Blake's passions was dress reform. In the spring of 1874, Blake, with homeopaths Caroline Hastings, Mercy B. Jackson, and Arvilla B. Haynes gave a series of five public lectures enumerating the physical disorders caused by layers of heavy skirts and tight lacing.[52] All were faculty members of the homeopathic medical college and had served at one time on the board of the WEIU. Many of their arguments against prevailing fashions were similar to those espoused by women regular physicians, who noted that while women's restrictive clothing caused physical damage, it also symbolized women's social and intellectual impotence or helplessness.[53] No evidence has been found showing that women regulars connected dress reform to class divisions hindering women's advancement, however. Hoping to broaden awareness of how women's personal decisions affected the good of all women, Boston homeopaths directed their appeal to the wealthy who, by their influence and example, promoted the "false burdens of fashion," perpetuating symbols of women's passivity in society. And, they argued, in their desire to emulate the "respectable" dress of wealthy, and upper- middle-class women, poor working girls suffered economic as well as physical consequences. Not only did the seamstress spend her days in sedentary confinement at her sewing machine producing finery for upper-class women, but she also sewed all night to create clothes for herself to appear respectable in the presence of elegantly-clothed customers. Middle-class women, unable to afford dressmakers, but anxious to seem wealthier than they were, sewed their own clothes,

leading their families into financial ruin with the purchase of cloth and acces-
sories enabling them to emulate upper-class standards.[54]

Within the rhetoric of dress reform as a means to better individual
health, women homeopaths revealed their own notions of the meaning of
republican nationhood, where there were "no distinct class lines so tightly
drawn that citizens cannot pass from one to the other." Understanding the
natural desires of the lower classes to elevate themselves, they encouraged
wealthy women to realize the consequences of their personal choices on their
less-favored sisters.[55]

Unlike Frances Janney, Anna Howard Shaw considered Mary Safford
Blake one of her "favorite" teachers. Calling her "a mite of a woman [another
source estimated Safford's height at four feet] with an indomitable soul,"
Shaw's admiration of Safford stemmed not only from the latter's indefatigable
medical work among Boston's poor and her extensive philanthropic efforts,
but also from Blake's activism on women's rights.[56] Anna Howard Shaw, an
ordained Methodist Episcopal minister by 1880, received a medical degree
from the homeopathic medical college at Boston University in 1885. She
became a prominent figure in the fight for women's political and social equality, and was a constant coworker and companion of Susan B. Anthony from
1888 to 1906. A nationally known lecturer on temperance and women's rights,
Dr. Shaw was president of Washington, D.C.'s Wimodaughsis in 1891; and in
1892, was elected vice president of the National American Woman Suffrage
Association (NAWSA). Beginning in 1904, she served as the organization's
president for eleven years. In later years, Shaw chaired the Women's Committee of the Council of National Defense. In 1919 President Woodrow Wilson
presented her with the Distinguished Service Medal for her longtime commitment to peace and women's rights through work in national and international
organizations.[57]

Mary Safford Blake also made a deep impression on Martha George Ripley, an 1883 graduate and classmate of Shaw's. Born in 1843 in Lowell, Vermont, Ripley was raised in a reform-minded family where her mother's
Freewill Baptist faith combined deep spirituality with a "resolute concern for
practical justice." Dedicated to the abolitionist cause, the family operated an
underground railroad station behind its home in Vermont before relocating to
the Iowa frontier in 1847. Martha George met her husband near Fort Atkin-
son following the Civil War. In 1867, the couple married and moved to
Lawrence, Massachusetts, where William Ripley ran his uncle's paper mill. In
the 1870s, after the birth of three daughters, Martha Ripley became active in
the American Woman Suffrage Association led by Lucy Stone and Julia Ward
Howe. But Ripley considered the organization's single-minded focus on na-

tional suffrage impractical. She observed that an abstract right such as "suffrage" had less meaning to women than being able to vote in local school elections or for temperance laws in their localities.[58]

During this time Ripley became a popular speaker on woman suffrage, and was elected to the executive committees of both the New England Woman Suffrage Association and the Massachusetts Woman Suffrage Association, forming lifelong friendships with prominent reformers. Her committee associates included homeopath Mercy B. Jackson and regular physician Marie E. Zakrzewska. After moving to Minneapolis in the early 1880s, Ripley was elected president of the Minnesota Woman Suffrage Association in 1883. Her home was a center for reformers active in suffrage, public health, and women's equal representation on the local board of education and police department. In a series of letters to Minneapolis newspapers, Ripley argued in favor of "matrons" on the Minneapolis police, the right of female domestics to unionize, and women's right to be elected to boards of education. A member of the Women's Rescue League, she led crusades to reform and rehabilitate the city's prostitutes; conducted a war on "filth" and battled for pure water; condemned food adulteration; and argued for more spacious and sanitary accommodations in the city hospital, thereby combining her work for women's equal rights under the law with moral and sanitary reform. Like Blake and Shaw, Ripley promoted cremation arguing that burial, not only endangered public health, but also imposed economic hardship on the "landless urban masses" unable to afford traditional internment. Ripley's most lasting legacy was the establishment of Maternity Hospital in Minneapolis with a medical department "under the care and control of homeopathic women physicians," and a board of directors comprised solely of women, including prominent women homeopaths, suffragists, school board candidates, and one lawyer. Until her death in 1915, Ripley was the heart and soul of the hospital.[59]

Social Class and Homeopathy

Women homeopaths in the vanguard of social reform activities tended to be socially prominent in their communities, reinforcing homeopathy's links with a growing and increasingly affluent middle class. Indeed, several scholars have shown that homeopathy made its greatest gains among the urban middle and upper classes.[60] A statistical analysis of Worcester and Suffolk Counties in Massachusetts from 1855 to 1875, showed that homeopaths occupied a higher socioeconomic position, serving more affluent patients than regular physicians.[61] In Philadelphia, elites patronizing homeopathy included "old money" families with names such as Strawbridge, Clothier, Widener, Wharton, and

Biddle.[62] In Rochester, New York, they included many of the city's "more recently prominent and prosperous citizens" such as Hiram Sibley, organizer of Western Union and the "richest man in town."[63] Cleveland homeopath Myra King Merrick, founder of Cleveland Homoeopathic Hospital and College for Women in 1868, was physician to John D. Rockefeller and "all the Standard Oil families"; and, the homeopathic practice of Stella Manning Perkins of Lynn, Massachusetts, included the prominent Spragues of Swampscott as well as other "leading families."[64]

While practicing homeopathic medicine in New York City in the 1870s, Anna Manning met and subsequently married George F. Comfort, a distinguished American art educator and founding trustee of the Metropolitan Museum of Art. When George Comfort was offered a deanship at the newly established Fine Arts College at Syracuse University around 1880, the couple moved to Syracuse, where Dr. Comfort established her medical practice and joined a variety of professional and reform organizations, including the Professional Woman's League of Syracuse, the Syracuse Political Equality Club, and the New York State Woman Suffrage Association. Through frequent letters and articles to local newspapers, she became well known for her defense of women's rights as well as those of American Indians and African Americans.[65] While these examples reveal the social prominence of women homeopaths in communities, their experiences as physicians also were influenced by their numerical parity with women regulars in specific areas.

According to William Rothstein, in 1898 homeopaths comprised only 8 percent of all practitioners in the United States.[66] The numerical marginality of homeopaths has contributed to the notion that homeopaths were viewed as the medical "other." More meaningful, however, is the number of homeopaths of each sex in particular cities and their percentages of the combined population of homeopaths and regulars. Statistics show that male homeopaths always comprised a small minority of the male physician populations in urban areas. This was not the case for women, however. As Appendix B shows, at different points in time and in particular locations, women homeopaths were equal to or more numerous than women regular practitioners. For example, Susan McKinney practiced in Brooklyn when women homeopaths were a majority of all women doctors in the city. A socially prominent, successful homeopath, McKinney's African American heritage further reinforced homeopathy's liberal image. Reporting on the March 23, 1870, graduation exercises of New York Medical College and the Hospital for Women, *The Courier*, described Susan Marie Smith (later McKinney) as "3/4 white" with "good features, charming black eyes, and soft, black, wavy ringlets." According to the paper, she was attired in black silk, with a large red ribbon knotted at her "finely arched neck," adding: "Miss Smith belongs to the colored aristocracy in Brooklyn and is a member of the Episcopal Church."[67] The seventh of ten children, Smith was born in Brooklyn's Weeksville section in 1847 to Sylvanus Smith, a prosperous hog farmer, and Anne Springsteel Smith. Her two sisters became schoolteachers, and Smith herself taught public school in Washington, D.C., for two years before settling on the more "progressive" career of medicine. Her longtime friend, Hallie Q. Brown, believed caring for her niece during an illness influenced Smith's decision to alleviate sickness and suffering on a broader scale. Although her family was prosperous, she took pride in her self-reliance, paying her own school expenses by teaching in a Manhattan "colored school."[68]

In 1871, she married William G. McKinney, a moderately wealthy clergyman from South Carolina. Shortly thereafter, she attended post-graduate courses at the regular Long Island College Hospital in Brooklyn. Throughout her forty-eight-year career, McKinney took an active part in her profession. In 1879 she became a member of Kings County Homoeopathic Medical Society and was an organizer of her alma mater's alumni society; in the 1880s, she presented papers at meetings of the Homeopathic Medical Society of New York. In 1881 she helped found the Brooklyn Woman's Homoeopathic Hospital and Dispensary and became a staff surgeon in 1891. She built her reputation and practice upon skillful treatment of children's diseases, specifically "marasmus" or malnutrition (characterized by vomiting and diarrhea thought to be caused by unsuitable food and "inherited" syphilis). McKinney firmly believed children suffering from marasmus and other diseases stood a "far better chance of recovery under homeopathic treatment."[69] Her successful career helped the couple to move into a large residence on Ryerson Street in Brooklyn. Located in a predominantly white neighborhood, the house eventually accommodated ten people, including the McKinney's two children and various relatives. In 1890 the family moved to DeKalb Avenue, described in the New York Times as "in the midst of the fashionable quarter of the hill."[70]

Similar to the experience of many women physicians at the time, McKinney's practice was slow in the beginning as people adjusted to the idea of patronizing a woman doctor. However, by 1900, her patients, both white and black, female and male, had made her a wealthy physician. The Brooklyn Daily Eagle of August 18, 1891, listed her among the city's "famous doctors." Another 1891 story in the Brooklyn Daily Times featured McKinney and four other prominent women physicians, noting that two-thirds of the city's female physicians were homeopathic doctors and that her varied practice included "the high, the low, the rich, and the poor." In a tribute to Brooklyn's prominent doctors, the Brooklyn Daily Times of June 17, 1891, called McKinney "the most successful practitioner of medicine of her sex and race in the United States."[71] And contributing to evidence that professional relations between homeopaths and regulars were often cordial, especially in the latter part of the century, the reporter noted that "it was an allopathic physician of highest standing who bade me by all means to see Dr. McKinney."[72]

Besides attending to her medical practice, McKinney was active in missionary work, education reform, temperance, and woman's suffrage. After the death of her husband in 1894, she married Reverend Theophilus Gould Steward in 1896, chaplain of the Twenty-fifth United States Colored Infantry. Her own children grown, she assumed responsibility for Steward's children. They eventually moved to Wilberforce, Ohio, where both she and her husband were appointed to the faculty of Wilberforce University, and she was resident physician. Her life included European travel and attendance at the First Universal Race Congress in London (July 1911), where W.E.B. Du Bois and other prominent Asians, Africans, Americans, and Europeans discussed ways to improve relationships between "so-called white and so-called colored peoples." Dr. McKinney Steward made sure that women were part of the conversation on race by delivering a paper on "Colored American Women" highlighting the achievements of such notable African American women as Phillis Wheatley, Ida Wells-Barnett, and Mary Church Terrell. She was equally concerned with issues of gender and race. Her 1914 paper on "Women in Medicine" delivered at the National Association of Colored Women's Clubs in Wilberforce argued against separate medical schools for women. The "great need," she said, was more internships and "equality of opportunity for hospital service."[73] Dr. McKinney Steward died on March 7, 1918. Her body was returned from Ohio to New York for funeral services. At the Brooklyn home of her daughter, eulogies for the respected doctor were delivered by William S. Scarborough, president of Wilberforce University, Dr. Helen S. Lassen, a former classmate, and prominent black leader and intellectual, W.E.B. Du Bois.

The Second Generation

Histories of the women's movement have chronicled the shifting alliances, priorities, and changing composition of groups over the course of the nineteenth century.[74] According to Gloria Moldow, the pioneer homeopaths of Washington, D.C.'s WEIU and Wimodaughsis were disappointed when their goals of cross-class female solidarity and commitment to feminism lacked appeal for the next generation of women physicians, leading to the demise of those organizations. A new generation, exemplified by Frances Janney, often disparaged early women activists, believing their tactics unseemly and their goals unsuitable to the altered professional milieu in which women doctors found themselves.[75] The coeducational experiment was largely considered a success, and women had gained access to most medical societies. Women had demonstrated their intellectual and physical ability to practice medicine, and Janney considered radicalism on the part of women in the profession inappropriate, unnecessary, and unprofessional. Although second-generation women physicians continued their support of suffrage, they also joined new organizations stimulated by the Progressive Era's interest in preventive medicine and sanitary reform. By the last decade of the century, women homeopaths and regulars began to bridge their professional partition.

During the last third of the nineteenth century, the homeopathic profession gradually distanced itself from its earlier association with social reform. As homeopaths discovered more ideological and professional similarities than differences with scientific medicine, they reexamined their profession's broadly defined antiorthodox identity.[76] The notion of orthodoxy itself was gradually replaced by an inclusive definition of science, and recognizing the pecuniary benefits of consultation, regular physicians lobbied against the AMA's code against consultation with irregulars and in some cases simply ignored it.[77] Liberalizing tendencies among regulars and homeopathy's changing identity refocused relations between the professions on similarities rather than differences. Women regular physicians, now less concerned that association with women homeopaths threatened their own professional status, joined a number of organizations whose members included women homeopaths. The WEIU in Boston, for example, was staffed exclusively with women homeopaths until the middle of the 1880s. But in 1889, even Marie Zakrewska who had distanced herself from any association with irregular medicine joined homeopath Julia M. Plummer as the organization's physician consultants.[78] When Carolyn Winslow founded the Washington, D.C., chapter of the WEIU around 1889, she succeeded in attracting both homeopathic and regular women physicians to the organization.[79] By the last decade of the century, women physicians of both schools of medicine recognized common interests as professional women and social leaders, and actively joined new types of women's organizations. The Daughters of the American Revolution (DAR), the Association of Collegiate Alumnae (later the American Association of University Women), and business women's clubs, among others, paralleled male-only organizations; like them, they reinforced women's professional middle-class identities, facilitated contacts that advanced their careers, and heightened their public esteem.[80]

Neurologist and homeopath Eliza Taylor Ransom was part of this new generation of women physicians. Ransom graduated from the homeopathic

Boston University School of Medicine in 1900. Establishing a practice in Boston, Ransom became famous for her leadership of the Twilight Sleep Movement in New England, founded the first twilight sleep hospital in the United States, and argued for women's right to choose pain-free labor and delivery. Her professional activities included membership in the Boston Homoeopathic Medical Society (1902) and the Massachusetts Homoeopathic Medical Society, where in 1905 she was elected first vice president. In 1901 she was professor of histology at Boston University School of Medicine; and in addition to her private practice, was employed by the Equitable Life Insurance Society of the United States as medical examiner for women. Ransom was a member of several in medical organizations as well as an inveterate clubwoman, belonging to numerous civic and professional women's organizations: the Women's City Club, the Business and Professional Women's Club, the Canadian Club of Boston, and the Copley Society of Boston, patronizing its musicales and recitals. Contemporary articles in local newspapers attest to Ransom's position in the upper echelons of Boston society, featuring her attendance at charity events, pouring at numerous teas, and serving on committees comprised of both homeopathic and regular physicians.[81] Ransom's suffrage activities included numerous speaking engagements at rallies throughout New England as well as locally, where she was Ward Eleven's representative to the Massachusetts Woman Suffrage Association. She ardently supported coeducation, and chose the subject for her speech to the graduating class of Boston's medical school in 1900. Reflecting her generation's optimism that women no longer required single-sex colleges as a means to medical education, she believed that women were recognized as equal and "complementary" to men in institutions of higher education.[82]

Missing from History

Although throughout the nineteenth and into the twentieth century, women homeopaths were leaders in various strands of the woman's movement as well as founders of medical schools and hospitals, their identities as homeopathic doctors have gone largely unrecognized. In 1974, Brooklyn's junior high school No. 265 was renamed the Dr. Susan Smith McKinney Junior High School; and in recent years, African American female physicians in New York, New Jersey, and Connecticut have named medical societies in her honor.[83] While both school children and African American female physicians know Susan McKinney Steward as a pioneer, surmounting obstacles of both race and gender in her chosen profession, few are aware of her identity as a homeopathic physician. Similarly, a recent Public Broadcasting Service documentary on woman suffrage titled "One Woman, One Vote," highlighted Anna Howard Shaw's leadership, referring to her as a "female doctor" and graduate of Boston University Medical College. Shaw's identity as a homeopath would be known only to those with knowledge of the history of medical institutions.

The absence of homeopathy as a defining characteristic in the lives of many women practitioners rests largely on how women homeopaths envisioned themselves and how they were viewed by the general public. Present-day studies that exclude women homeopaths from discussions of "women in medicine" or emphasize homeopathy's deviance from accepted medical theory and practice, often promote the false idea that a physician's identity as "homeopath" or "regular" was of overriding importance to themselves, their patients, and other doctors throughout the nineteenth century. Although an individual's medical affiliation was an important element in institutional cultures of medical schools, medical societies, and hospitals, more important for our purposes is how women conceived of themselves within a broader framework. Scholars' use of the terms "sectarian" and "irregular," pejorative terms describing homeopathy and its practitioners, mainly derive from inflammatory rhetoric in contemporary medical publications and articles written by doctors. Although patients' choice of homeopathy up to about 1860 evidenced their opposition to the debilitating therapeutics of regulars, it is doubtful the general public considered homeopaths "unorthodox" or "irregular" in the ways we have come to use and understand the terms. And by the time women entered the profession in significant numbers, everyday relations between average physicians of both schools were often quite congenial. Pioneer women homeopaths' descriptions of their early struggles suggest gender rather than medical ideology influenced patients' thinking. As pioneers in the medical profession, their experiences were similar to those of their sisters practicing regular medicine.

When Anna Manning Comfort established her first practice in Norwich, Connecticut, shortly after graduating in 1865, she was taunted in the streets, and her medical sign was removed repeatedly from her home office—not because she was a homeopath, but because she attempted to enter a male domain professionally. In 1886 Sarah J. Millsop, a northerner and self-described "homoeopathist," moved to Bowling Green, Kentucky, where the presence of a "woman doctor" was almost unheard of. Although the city was an "Allopathic stronghold," Millsop placed notices of her new practice in both local papers, and within a week had "thrown my 'shingle' to the breeze." At first, she was such a curiosity that people in the street often turned to look at her, exclaiming: "There goes the woman doctor!" But within a month, Millsop drew patients not only from Bowling Green but also from adjoining towns and even other states, noting: "Ladies from Mississippi and Tennessee have told me that women doctors were greatly needed in those States; many women having to go away from home for Gynaecological treatment." Millsop's identity as a homeopath seemed important to only a few. For example, two families from the lower South contemplating spending the summer in Bowling Green would not finalize their plans for lodging until they ascertained the presence of a local homeopathic doctor. But to most of Millsop's patients, long accustomed to heroic doses of drugs, she was simply the "lady doctor [who] don't give strong medicine."[84]

By 1879 homeopath Sofia Penfield had practiced medicine in Danbury, Connecticut, for seven years. In a country town of ten thousand residents, Penfield was the only woman among nine physicians, all but one, "old school practitioners." According to Penfield, when she first began her practice, prejudice against women physicians was so strong that "the Doctors refused me consultation or assistance; but that has worn away. They now treat me with respect and are willing to render me any assistance in the way of a consultation, that can be held between the two schools." And after seven years, she noted: "My practice is good, comprising some of the most influential and intelligent families in the town."[85]

In cities such as Boston where battles between homeopaths and regulars were publicly fought, it is likely that physicians strongly identified with their respective professions, prohibiting cooperative relationships between physicians as noted by Penfield. In urban areas where patients could choose from various practitioners, some patronized only doctors of a particular school, but most switched back and forth between doctors searching for cures. In rural areas underserved by women physicians of either school, whether a doctor was regular or homeopathic was often less important than gender. In Sara Milsop's experience, the most significant characteristic of her practice to patients was her disdain of strong medicine.

The conflation of the two professions in the mind of the public after the turn of the century presents problems for the historian seeking to distinguish homeopaths from regulars. When prominent Philadelphia homeopath Harriet French died of a stroke in September 1906, over three hundred mourners paid their respects to the woman who had been president of the Philadelphia County Women's Christian Temperance Union (WCTU) for fifty years. A Philadelphia newspaper noted that French was "the second woman to receive a doctor's degree from a Philadelphia institution" and "the oldest woman doctor in the city." It chronicled her work in temperance, curfew laws for children, the prevention of cruelty to animals, and other reforms, but did not indicate French had been a homeopath.[86] In an article titled "Minnesota Memories," appearing in the *Minneapolis Tribune* in 1948, Martha G. Ripley was called a "pioneer woman physician, founder of Maternity Hospital in Minneapolis." The author noted that Ripley had always felt the urge to "become a physician," and that she had graduated from the "Boston University medical school" with full honors before heading west to Minneapolis.[87] Anna Manning Comfort repeatedly referred to herself as a "regularly graduated medical woman."[88] An 1896 article in the *Syracuse Post* about Comfort and her devotion to the "profession of medicine" noted that when she graduated in 1865, "there were not over a dozen regular women meical graduates in America."[89] And in an 1895 article highlighting the city's prominent women in the professions of law, medicine, and the ministry, Comfort was called the "earliest woman medical graduate in this city . . . [and] . . . the first woman to break the conservative medical ranks in staid Connecticut," the location of her first practice.[90] In her 1915 autobiography, Anna Howard Shaw said she obtained her medical diploma from "Boston Medical School" and became a "full-fledged physician," making no mention of homeopathy.[91] Perhaps Shaw saw no need to identify her graduating institution as homeopathic, as it would have been common knowledge at the time.[92] Shaw's description of herself is that of a doctor whose primary concern was to alleviate suffering and cure disease among the poor in tenements lining the alleys of Maiden's Lane, Fellows Court, and Andrews Court in Boston.

Perhaps Comfort and Shaw sought to distance themselves from their "irregular" past, neglecting to mention what historians perceive as their most distinguishing characteristic. But Shaw's autobiography was published three years before the medical school at BU abolished its connection with homeopathy. In writing about her alma mater, fellow students, and professors, Shaw was not trying to hide her homeopathic identity. Comfort's use of the term "regularly educated physician," was one she used early in her career. She was not denying her homeopathic affiliation, but emphasizing the most essential aspect of her identity—that of a woman doctor whose graduate institution was fully chartered by the State of New York and equal to the best medical schools of the time.

Womens' decision to emphasize their affiliation with homeopathic medicine around the turn of the century and later, depended upon whether a homeopathic identity was useful or detrimental to professional goals. Women with high social standing and secure practices, living in areas where women homeopaths were equal in number to women regulars, did not consider their association with homeopathic medicine a disadvantage. Physicians such as

Sarah Millsop, Anna Howard Shaw, Mary Safford Blake, Martha Ripley, Anna Manning Comfort, among others, considered themselves "regular" doctors in the fullest sense of the word. The numerical superiority of women homeopaths in particular cities, their successful practices, high social status, prominent clientele, and the women's descriptions of themselves as doctors leads to a new understanding of what it meant to be a woman homeopathic practitioner. Rather than marginal to American medicine, they were an integral part of it.

Chapter 3   Becoming Physicians

Women's Homeopathic Medical Education, 1852–1900

In August of 1874, Frances Janney left her home in Columbus, Ohio, to serve a medical apprenticeship under the guidance of two male homeopathic physicians in Indianapolis—Drs. Hunt and Runnels. In a letter to her parents soon after beginning her studies, Janney said she was studying the bones, nerves, and muscles of the head. Perhaps as a way of illustrating that she possessed the intestinal fortitude necessary to become a physician, she casually informed them that she was using a human skull "that is supposed to have belonged to a rebel prisoner."[1]

Janney found both doctors "very kind," and especially liked Dr. Runnels's "interesting impromptu lectures . . . [and] ideas about studying." Janney intended to apply for admission to a medical college in the fall of 1874 after learning the basics of anatomy and physiology from Hunt and Runnels. She informed her parents that Dr. Hunt "wants me to know a little more than any of the men for a woman has enough to contend with anyway." According to Janney, she and her preceptors weighed the pros and cons of several homeopathic medical schools before deciding on the homeopathic medical college at Boston University.[2]

At first glance, Janney's choice of a homeopathic school seems to support the idea that sectarian medical colleges provided women with the opportunity for medical education at a time when regular medical colleges refused to admit them. Yet it does not necessarily follow that most women entered homeopathic colleges through lack of options, even during the pioneer years of women in medicine. Nor does it suggest that male homeopaths held more liberal views of women's medical education at that time. Like women regular physicians prior to 1870, most women homeopaths attended women's medical schools. By founding separate homeopathic colleges in Cleveland and New York, women created their own early opportunities for homeopathic training.[3] After 1870, when opportunities for both regular and homeopathic coeducation expanded, the numbers of women choosing homeopathic schools increased substantially.[4]

Francis Janney was one of approximately sixteen hundred women graduates of homeopathic colleges by the turn of the century; and between 1890 and 1900, they represented 18 percent of all homeopathic college graduates. Although the vast majority of women entered regular medical schools during the final decades of the century, those who became homeopaths considered themselves legitimate physicians—not unorthodox practitioners. Women's homeopathic education conformed in kind and quality to that of women in the regular profession. Women considered their training in homeopathic therapeutics an added benefit, not a substitute or replacement for the latest medical knowledge.

Women's Early Education

When Helen Cook and Frances Woodruff graduated from the Western College of Homoeopathic Medicine in Cleveland in 1852, women were a rarity in America's medical schools.[5] Although a few were enrolled with men in eclectic schools in New York, Massachusetts, and Pennsylvania, only two all-female regular schools matriculated women: New England Female Medical College in Boston, and the Female Medical College of Pennsylvania (later the Woman's Medical College of Pennsylvania).[6]

The curriculum of Cook and Woodruff's homeopathic medical school was typical of most homeopathic and regular colleges of the day, offering didactic lectures in surgery, anatomy, materia medica, chemistry, and physical science.[7] Students attended two years of lectures; the second term was a repetition of the first. Fees for each year's instruction totaled $99, and the school was heavily dependent upon tuition income. The decision in 1850 to admit women to Western College of Homoeopathic Medicine in Cleveland appears to have served the school's pecuniary interest, and was influenced by liberal faculty members.[8] After a faculty reorganization in 1863, however, more conservative voices prevailed. Opponents to women's education argued that women lowered the "scientific standard" of the college.[9] They believed the school's reputation would be enhanced by the absence of women, thus increasing the numbers of male applicants. In 1867, the registrar of the college sent a note to each woman student, requesting her withdrawal. After protesting that the faculty had struck a deathblow to women's medical education in Cleveland, women homeopaths there immediately organized to gather support for a women's college.[10]

Led by Cleora Seaman, an 1860 graduate of Western College of Homoeopathy, and homeopath Eliza King Merrick, an 1852 graduate of Central Eclectic Medical College in Rochester, New York, they founded the Cleveland Homoeopathic Hospital College for Women in the fall of 1867. Seaman served as president of the board of trustees, and Merrick was professor of obstetrics and diseases of women and children. Corresta T. Canfield, professor of anatomy, was the only other woman on the faculty with nine men. By all accounts, the training women received at the new institution was similar to that at the men's college. Besides sharing faculty, the two schools used similar textbooks, and both required attendance at two courses of lectures in the standard subjects. Merrick and Seaman arranged for their students' clinical work at Cleveland's City Hospital Infirmary.[11]

In 1869, trustees and faculty of the men's college embarked upon a campaign to solicit students throughout the West. Tuition funds were sorely needed to finance annual payments on a newly purchased college building and hospital. Expansion of the men's school required the goodwill of the community—especially women volunteers and fund-raisers—to establish a college hospital. And, as the women's college had been surprisingly successful—attracting forty-five students during its first three years—the faculty began to rethink its prohibition against women students. In 1869, Seth R. Beckwith—the most vociferous opponent of women's admission—resigned to accept a position at Cincinnati's Pulte Medical College, where he became a prominent opponent of that school's coeducation initiative a few years later.[12] Absent women's most influential and outspoken opponent, and in light of increased debt, the faculty of Western Homoeopathic College passed a resolution in 1870 stating, "there shall never hereafter be made any distinction in regard to sex, color, nationality, or religion" in the admission of students to matriculation and graduation.[13] Trustees and faculty of the college urged women to return, promising that "no distinction will be made in matriculation, course of instruction, or graduation." And, "All subjects best taught apart will be so given, thus avoiding the objections heretofore urged against medical education of the sexes."[14] Although Merrick and others opposed the union of the two schools, believing the board of the women's college acted illegally in transferring college property to the men's school, the merger went forward. In 1871 the combined institution was renamed Cleveland Homoeopathic Hospital College.

Although the Western College of Homoeopathy distinguished itself from regular male-only medical schools by its early admission of women, the school's uneven commitment resulted in relatively few women graduates during its first twenty years. More important to women's early homeopathic medical education, were institutions that women founded by and for themselves.[15] The most important institution in the history of women in homeopathic medicine was the New York Medical College and Hospital for Women (NYMCHW), founded in 1863 by reformer and women's rights activist, Clemence Lozier. The NYMCHW is notable, not only for the number of women graduates over its forty-five-year history (approximately 370 by 1914), but also for its leading role in raising the standards of medical education.

Clemence Lozier and the New York Medical College and Hospital for Women

As president and dean of NYMCHW until her death in 1888, Clemence Lozier presided over a faculty initially consisting of four women and four men, including nationally known New York homeopaths Timothy Field Allen and Carroll Dunham. Lecture subjects included: diseases of women and children; pathology and principles and practice of medicine; anatomy; obstetrics and medical jurisprudence; clinical and operative surgery; materia medica and diseases of the chest; and chemistry and toxicology. In their senior year, students received surgical and obstetrical practice under the supervision of professors, participated in oral and written discussions of medical topics, and, in the presence of professors and other students, advanced pupils diagnosed and treated patients' pathological conditions.[16] In 1864, the state legislature authorized the establishment of a hospital for women and children in connection with the college. An all-female board of trustees, including Elizabeth Cady Stanton, managed both the college and the hospital. Within a decade, the hospital averaged 150 patients and treated about 3,000 "sick poor" annually.[17]

The NYMCHW pioneered in supporting higher educational standards for students and in securing adequate clinical opportunities for women. Prior to the 1869–1870 session, trustees strengthened graduation requirements. Rather than repeating the same course of lectures for two successive terms (the standard at most medical schools), the new requirements specified three progressive courses of lectures, each five months in duration, with dissections mandated in the first and second years.[18] The requirements predated those adopted by such prestigious schools as Harvard Medical College and the University of Pennsylvania.[19] Most medical colleges in New York did not follow suit until as late as 1891. In fact, with the exception of the Woman's Medical

College of the New York Infirmary founded by Elizabeth Blackwell, educational standards at Lozier's homeopathic college exceeded those of most other regular medical schools for women until the turn of the century.

Five years after Lozier's founded NYMCHW, Elizabeth Blackwell established the city's first regular medical college for women. It is entirely possible that the competition between these two institutions to provide women with exemplary medical training, drove both to excel. Both schools introduced curricular innovations around the same time, requiring a three-year, progressive, graded curriculum in 1868. And the first course in hygiene (preventive medicine) offered anywhere in the country was listed in each of their 1868–1869 college catalogs. In 1893, the two institutions simultaneously lengthened their programs to four years. Along with the regular Woman's Medical College of Pennsylvania, both New York schools actively sought to increase clinical opportunities for female medical students—one of the most difficult challenges facing female medical students.[20]

Most medical education consisted of four to six hour-long lectures a day, five days a week. Once or twice a week students went to a local hospital where they walked the wards or watched surgeons perform autopsies and surgeries in an amphitheater filled with two or three hundred other students and physicians.[21] Although the dispensary and hospital associated with NYMCHW offered some clinical work, Lozier sought additional opportunities for women students. Learning that students at any accredited medical institution had the legal right to attend clinical lectures at state hospitals, she secured tickets of admission to several of the city's hospital clinics. However, women students seeking to attend such lectures were often harassed and intimidated by intolerant male students.

One incident took place in the late 1860s when trustee Elizabeth Cady Stanton accompanied a group of thirty women from the NYMCHW to Bellevue Hospital. She recalled that the women were "greeted by a thousand students with shouts of derisive laughter . . . pelted with chewed balls of paper . . . [and subjected by professors to] . . . the most offensive subject and disease for the day."[22] Soon after the incident, Lozier called a "public indignation meeting" at Cooper Institute to denounce the outrageous conduct of male students and the inaction of Bellevue's faculty in controlling their boorish behavior. Speakers included Horace Greeley, Henry Ward Beecher, and other prominent social reformers. With public opinion and the city's press siding with the women, the mayor of New York agreed to send a marshal and police force to the clinics to "protect the ladies in their rights."[23]

Lozier's struggle for women's equality was waged from within her institution as well. According to Stanton, Lozier exhibited great strength and perseverance in maintaining control of the college when its success caused "men . . . [to become] . . . most pertinacious in their attentions, and . . . determined to dominate her and the funds she raised to carry out her projects." Lacking qualified female professors in the college's early years, the board of trustees invited several professors of New York Homoeopathic College to teach in the women's school. But when Lozier tried to replace the men with competent women professors, some were reluctant to leave. In 1866, Isaac M. Ward refused to relinquish his position as professor of obstetrics when Lozier wanted to replace him with Anna Inman. According to Stanton, "it took us a whole year to oust the male professor . . . [because his] . . . influence over the board prevented us from having a quorum." After numerous board meetings, Lozier and Stanton traveled to Albany, presenting the "woman's side of the question" to the regents of the University of the State of New York. They returned with a decision in their favor, and Ward was released from his duties at the college.[24]

In a later incident, Lozier's ideas of sound institutional mangement conflicted with male advisers. Along with the board of trustees, decisions affecting the college were influenced by an advisory council consisting of local businessmen and faculty of the men's school. Although the college and hospital had prospered for twelve years at the corner of Second Avenue and Twelfth Street and was debt free, advisers proposed purchasing land at 301 Lexington Avenue to construct a new college and hospital buildings. According to Stanton, ". . . certain male professors in the institution, desiring larger buildings uptown, persuaded the women, with fair promises of aid, to sell out . . ."[25] Lozier strenuously opposed the move, but was overruled. In addition to the heavily mortgaged land, funds had to be raised for construction just when the nation suffered a severe financial collapse in 1873. According to Lozier's son, the panic of Black Friday spread a "dark cloud" over his mother's affairs. In the ensuing depression, the school's equity was depleted and friends, wealthy patrons, and advisers who had promised funds for the new construction "deserted" her.[26] Lozier lost her life savings when she could not cover a large number of bonds unexpectedly called in for payment, and in 1878, at the age of sixty-four, was forced into bankruptcy. Trustees abandoned plans for erecting costly buildings on Lexington Avenue and sold the property. The school struggled along, leasing temporary but inadequate quarters at Lexington Avenue and Thirty-seventh Street. But in 1881, invigorated in part by generous support from the newly-founded alumnae association, the board leased new and "commodious" buildings on West Fifty-fourth Street which was home to the school and hospital for the next twenty years.[27]

When Phoebe J. Wait was elected dean after Clemence Lozier's death in 1888, she remarked upon the changes in the student body since the school's inception. Whereas many earlier students were married women with little preliminary education who had tried other vocations and turned to medicine as a last resort, the current college boasted of students "in the bloom of life . . . fresh from college and full of enthusiasm."[28] Clinical opportunities were available at Ward's Island Hospital, the homeopathic New York Ophthalmic Hospital, the Laura Franklin Free Hospital for Children, Deaconess Institute of the Methodist Episcopal Church, and at numerous dispensaries throughout the city.[29]

In 1893, trustees and faculty required a four-year graded course, several years before its adoption by the majority of leading medical colleges. Sixteen professors and eleven lecturers, both men and women, taught all the standard medical subjects of the day, in addition to the homeopathic materia medica. In 1897 the college again upgraded its facilities, erecting a new building on 101st Street, west of Central Park. With generous support from New York's elite, William B. Tuthill, architect of Carnegie Hall, designed the new building. The modern structure contained a dispensary, lecture rooms, faculty offices, library, and laboratories fully equipped for histological, pathological, and bacteriological work. The adjoining hospital boasted the latest in modern appliances, including an electric elevator connecting the various levels to the spacious operating amphitheater on the top floor. At the end of the century, NYMCHW was one of the most up-to-date institutions of its kind and a fitting legacy to its founder.[30]

Despite their similar social status and professional goals for women in medicine, Clemence Lozier and Elizabeth Blackwell remained a world apart. Blackwell's contempt for sectarian practitioners was especially pointed toward Lozier. And while her hostility stemmed partly from being "upstaged," Blackwell also criticized Lozier's activism in radical reform movements—behavior she considered detrimental to women's overall advancement in the medical profession. Although woman's rights activist Susan B. Anthony chose homeopaths as her personal physicians, she desperately sought to bridge the gap separating Blackwell and Lozier: "It has been our most earnest desire to see these two institutions combined . . . and to this end we shall still labor."[31] But the two schools remained separate; and according to one source, Blackwell and Lozier ended their lives with an "icy gulf" between them.[32] And while Elizabeth Blackwell became a familiar figure in histories of women in medicine, Clemence Lozier is relatively unknown. Yet, NYMCHW graduated more than two hundred women by the end of the nineteenth century, nurturing the earliest generation of homeopathic practitioners and educators in an atmosphere of reform stimulated by the school's founder.

Although Blackwell disapproved of Lozier, the latter's reputation as a reformer may have increased the appeal of her school for many women. Anna

Manning, Clemence Lozier's niece, was a member of the first class to graduate from Lozier's college in 1865. During her school years, Manning resided with her aunt, who was also her preceptor. Susan B. Anthony, a frequent guest at her aunt's home, inspired Manning in her battles as a pioneer woman physician. Lozier's principles and activism also had a profound influence on the young woman, who at twenty years of age was one of the youngest graduates of the school. Manning considered her aunt "heroic," and took pride in the school's liberal reputation. She recalled her graduation ceremony, where she was escorted to the podium to receive her diploma by Horace Greeley and accompanied back to her seat by Henry Ward Beecher. Other notable reformers attended the celebration, lending support to women in medicine by their appearance and speeches, including Wendell Phillips, Julia Ward Howe, Susan B. Anthony, Lucretia Mott, Elizabeth Cady Stanton, William Lloyd Garrison, and Parker Pillsbury. Manning called it "a rallying occasion by the friends of women in medicine."[33]

Susan Smith McKinney began her studies at Lozier's college in 1867—just a few months prior to the July 1868 opening of Blackwell's school.[34] One historian suggests the homeopathic college was a natural selection because it allowed McKinney to live in her sister Sarah's Manhattan home while attending. However, the two schools were equally convenient to Sarah's home. More likely, McKinney chose Lozier's school because of its homeopathic teachings and/or Lozier's reputation as a reformer, especially her antiracism activities. McKinney's admission occasioned no protest from either students or faculty, and Clemence Lozier became Susan Smith McKinney's lifelong mentor and friend.[35]

Homeopathic Coeducation

Several historians have rightly questioned the assumption that homeopathic colleges eagerly welcomed women—that they ardently espoused sexual equality. In their study of coeducation at Cincinnati's homeopathic Pulte Medical College, William Barlow and David Powell show that the controversy over women's admission practically tore the school apart.[36] Two of the largest and most prestigious homeopathic medical colleges remained firmly closed to women throughout the nineteenth century. Hahnemann Medical College of Philadelphia, the largest homeopathic school in the country, rejected several appeals by women homeopaths in Pennsylvania for women's access to the college. And New York Homoeopathic Medical College refused to matriculate women until 1918, arguing women in New York already had access to homeopathic education at the New York Medical College and Hospital for Women.

Some distinguished homeopaths agreed with Harvard professor Edward H. Clarke, who popularized the idea that women would be subject to menstrual disability and reproductive disorders by attempting to conform to the routines and structure of schools developed for males.[37] Tullio Suzzara Verdi, a homeopathic specialist in obstetrics and gynecology in Washington, D. C., and president of the city's Board of Health in 1876, agreed with Clarke's thesis. Verdi published his conclusions in a popular health manual for mothers and daughters, warning that coeducation caused "overexertion" of the intellect, predisposing women to uterine and ovarian diseases.[38] Student theses often reflected similar notions. Frank F. Laird, a student at Hahnemann Medical College of Philadelphia, cited coeducation as a "powerful factor in producing disease" in women, endangering the welfare of the race as a whole.[39] And regular physicians were not alone in their concerns that women's "improper exposures" in coeducational lecture halls and clinics would destroy their "natural female modesty and refinement."[40] By 1880, however, nine out of eleven homeopathic colleges admitted women.[41] Since the majority of homeopathic schools were proprietary institutions, we can speculate that the pecuniary interests of colleges took precedence over the personal biases of individual physicians. In some cases evidence supports this hypothesis.

Administrators of Hahnemann Medical College in Philadelphia rejected appeals to admit women at a time when faculty, as a group, agreed to pledge $6,000 per year to support a hospital in conjunction with the college. Trustees wished to avoid "any experiment that may jeopardize our ability to accomplish this."[42] Amos Russell Thomas, dean of Hahnemann's faculty from 1874 to 1895, refused several petitions for women's admission presented over the years by the Women's Homoeopathic Medical Club of Philadelphia. While acknowledging women's importance to the profession, the faculty feared a drop in financial support from benefactors, and the flight of male students unwilling to study with females.[43]

In his 1886 response to members of the Women's Homoeopathic Medical Club of Philadelphia, Dean A. R. Thomas wrote: "We realize that the trend of public sentiment favors it [coeducation], especially is this manifested by those who do not intend to become students of medicine."[44] Fearing a loss of status, a decline in the number of male applicants, and withheld support by alumni, Hahnemann did not admit women until 1941 when World War II severely curtailed the number of male applicants.

In some places, women's admission may have aided the financial interests of schools. Founded in 1861, Hahnemann Medical College of Chicago (HMCC) opened its door to women in 1871, coinciding with the purchase of new college and hospital buildings. Perhaps as in Cleveland, faculty and trustees believed liberal policies regarding women students would spur the interest and generosity of laywomen in fund-raising activities on behalf of the institution. But a combination of interests was more likely responsible for coeducational policies of homeopathic colleges, including a sincere dedication to women's equal opportunity by several leaders in the profession.

Ruben Ludlam, a founder of Hahnemann Medical College of Chicago and its dean for twenty-five years beginning in 1866, championed women's equal educational and professional opportunity within homeopathy. Ludlam, a leading proponent of women's admission to the American Institute of Homoeopathy in the late 1860s, influenced colleagues on the faculty and board of trustees of HMCC to adopt coeducation in 1871.[45] Around the same time in Boston, a combination of influential liberal male homeopaths, pecuniary interests, and women's activism resulted in women's admission to Boston University School of Medicine, New England's first coeducational medical school.

While homeopaths in Boston negotiated with Boston University (BU) to organize a homeopathic medical college, the Massachusetts Medical Society expelled all "irregular" members, including eight prominent homeopaths who were long-standing members of the organization. One of the outcasts, Israel Talbot, was a Harvard graduate and personal physician to many prominent Bostonians, including Isaac Rich, a founder of Boston University. From 1871 to 1873, their "trial" and expulsion elicited outrage from the press, which berated the regulars for their petty, punitive actions. Much public sympathy lay with the ousted homeopaths, resulting in a surge of financial support for the new Massachusetts Homoeopathic Hospital and the rapid growth of the hospital's Ladies Aid Association. Women in Boston raised substantial sums for the new homeopathic hospital through two fund-raising fairs in 1870 and 1872. Feminists also urged homeopaths not to exclude women from the new college, reminding them of the additional pecuniary support they could expect from women, both as students and as fund-raisers.[46]

Boston was home to several prominent advocates of homeopathy including Louisa May Alcott, Julia Ward Howe, and Elizabeth Stuart Phelps. In a letter to *The New England Medical Gazette* in January 1873, Phelps urged organizers of the new school to "start right upon the education of women." Such a decision, she assured the *Gazette's* readers, would double the "instructive" and "pecuniary" forces of the college—a result of increased public interest, patronage, and respect." Several of the school's founders supported coeducation, including Israel Talbot, first dean of the new college, David Thayer, a prominent member of the Massachusetts legislature, and Conrad Wesselhoeft, nationally known for his contribution to homeopathic literature.[47]

Lacking a suitable facility for the new enterprise, trustees of Boston University entered into negotiations with trustees of the faltering New England Female Medical College. In addition to land, buildings, and equipment, the school controlled substantial endowments. Trustees voted to transfer the property to BU, provided the new owners agreed to maintain the college in accordance with its charter whose main provision was the medical education of women.[48]

Although coeducation at BU did not emerge from a singular commitment to equal opportunity for women, trustees and faculty expressed pride in the school's reputation for reform—both in its high educational standards and the abolition of all "sex disabilities in teaching and learning."[49] Out of an entering class of forty-three students, twenty were women. Mercy B. Jackson, Mary Safford Blake, and Caroline Hastings were among the original twenty-six member faculty.

The homeopathic medical school at BU was one of the largest of its kind in the country, and according to many homeopaths, one of the best. In the 1870s, the college led in instituting educational reforms—raising admission requirements, lengthening terms of study, adding new subjects to the curriculum, and shifting from didactic lectures to clinical experience.[50] From its founding in 1874, the homeopathic school instituted a three-year graded program, requiring either a bachelor of arts degree or successful performance on an entrance exam for admission. In 1878 the lecture term was extended from five to eight months; and in 1890, the school instituted a four-year graded course. Laboratory instruction was part of the curriculum, including some of the earliest laboratory exercises in pharmacology. Students conducted drug provings in medical and pharmaceutical chemistry and materia medica courses. In the late 1870s, Conrad Wesselhoeft, professor of materia medica and therapeutics, was among the first to institute the use of control groups and placebos in drug testing.[51] By 1893, laboratory courses included histology, physiology, pathological anatomy, surgery, and first-year studies of chemistry, physics, zoology, botany, and microscopy.

The early experiences of women at regular medical coeducational institutions have been well documented by historians. They tolerated social ostracism, deliberate animosity, and the boorish behavior of male students because they believed they would receive an education superior to what female-only colleges offered.[52] Yet, little is known about women's experiences in homeopathic schools. How were they treated by male faculty and students? What was their impression of professors, classmates, and the quality of education? Frances Janney attended BU from 1874 to 1877, a member of the first class to graduate from the medical school. She wrote daily to her parents and sister in

Columbus, Ohio. Her letters provide some insight into the social and academic culture at BU, as well as Janney's sense of herself as a woman and a homeopathic practitioner.

Frances Janney—Boston University Medical Student (1874–1876)

Frances Janney's Quaker parents, John Jay and Rebecca Smith Janney, were committed to women's rights and supported their daughter's decision to study medicine. After moving east to attend the homeopathic medical college at Boston University, Janney secured lodging at the boarding house of Mercy Jackson, a professor of women's diseases at the school. On the morning of October 7, 1874, Janney entered the large, new lecture room at the college to hear welcoming speeches by the school's president, Professor De Gersedorff, and Dean Israel Talbot. "The Professors," she noted, "are a fine looking set of men," and as the only female present at the lecture, Janney said the male students had a "good chance to look at me." She was gratified to hear Professor de Geredorff state that "With the exception of a few college graduates, the women who have entered here have a much better preparatory education than the men," implying that only a few students—mostly men—entered with bachelor of arts degrees.[53]

Janney's first-year studies included anatomy, physiology, botany, chemistry, and microscopy. In subsequent years, she studied ophthalmology, surgery and surgical pathology, diseases of children, gynecology, obstetrics, general practice, pathology and diagnostics, and homeopathic materia medica and therapeutics. Although first-year students were required to attend anatomical demonstrations every day, dissections were often stymied by the lack of subjects. "People won't die to order," she wrote.[54] In the spring of 1875, new microscopes arrived. Janney called them "splendid instruments," and at $45 hoped to have one herself some day. Janney encouraged her mother to inform John Grifith—an uncle who apparently believed his niece's decision to become a doctor would be undermined by the realities of the task—that she had "been a witness of the most disagreeable sights in the dissecting room and have nearly come to the bone in the arm I am working upon . . . [yet] . . . I have not the least idea of backing out."[55] Her schedule generally consisted of five lectures a day in classes with both male and female students, where she took notes and later recopied them in ink to "study them up."[56] But Janney believed her clinical experience was insufficient: "I want practical knowledge so badly and it is impossible to gain it here. They have a great many patients in the dispensary but it does not amount to much to me, for I cannot leave my lectures to go there."[57]

By the middle of her second year, her head was "in a whirl" from her studies, but she knew she was making progress. "I am beginning to understand different diseases, and the light is breaking on the method of curing them."[58] Final exams for the year began in February 1876. She received a grade of "80" in ophthalmology, "not very high, but still quite fair," considering sixteen in the class did not pass and only two students got perfect scores. Professor Mary Safford Blake's exam in gynecology began at 4:30 P.M. on February 13, and it was after 8:00 P.M. when Janney had answered the thirty-six exam questions and returned home, "completely exhausted." "We have three exams this week then I may take one more." After that, Janney planned to return home for the summer.[59]

On December 24, 1876, Janney and fellow student Abbie Rollins began writing their theses together at Rollins's home. They completed them in six days; Janney's subject was human parasites and Rollins's was pneumonia. Janney complained in a letter home that the thesis was a waste of time, inherently lacking originality because of students' inadequate practical experience and insufficient time to investigate theories or read thoroughly any one subject.[60] She thought the thesis requirement was a "farce" and "all nonsense" for it only shows "that we have access to books."[61] Janney worried that Professor De Gersdorff, who reviewed hers, would "pick it to pieces!" But deGersdorff gave her a "pretty good" mark, saying that the "ladies were much better than the gentlemen," and that "he *could not* accept" some of the latter.[62]

In January, Janney described her last months at the college. Students were called upon in groups of six (four "gentlemen" and two "ladies") to prepare patients for Saturday operations. In a letter to her sister Anne, Janney described how she etherized a patient with a sponge in front of an amphitheater full of students—many from Harvard—but "I did not care a bit." Dr. Jennegan asked her some questions "but he did not catch me." Janney said as she stood there before all the students she thought of the "trouble in New York" over women's admission to clinics, noting how "different" it was in the Boston hospitals.[63] She worried about her upcoming performance the following week when she would be required to perform an amputation "before the whole class on a cadaver." And yet, she was mastering the necessary art of emotional restraint: "I know I shall ligate (sic) a nerve or do something else ridiculous; and yet they all think me very cool and collected about anything I am obliged to do . . . I am glad I do not show my feelings."[64]

Janney's letters describe a medical education consisting of all the standard medical subjects of the day. Textbooks used in courses were authored by homeopathic as well as regular physicians, and Janney's lecture notes in obstetrics, physiology, and gynecology reflect teachings common to the regular school of medicine. Her education emphasized knowledge of the basic sciences, pathology, technological aids to diagnosis, and proficiency in surgical procedures—standard elements of medical education at comparable regular schools. For her, homeopathic principles and practice were additional tools to diagnose and treat disease; and she considered the study of materia medica one of her most difficult subjects. In a letter to her father, Janney wrote: "My bug-bear this year is going to be materia medica. The moment a professor mentions any remedies, I wilt."[65]

Throughout Janney's correspondence with family members, she frequently mentioned homeopathic remedies. During a summer under the tutelage of her preceptor Dr. Hunt, Janney wrote of her sympathy for a neighbor's child, a three-month-old baby who had the "flux" and whose "cries and moans" were constant. ". . . the poor young mother kneels by the cradle and watches every movement. I hardly think it can get well, especially as they have an allopathic doctor."[66] In Boston, Janney wrote of Mr. Mason, an occupant in the home in which she boarded:

> He came to me for some 'sugar pils' the other day, because he drank
> too much champagne. I was at my desk writing and the medicine was
> right before me, but I refused to give him any . . . He wanted to know
> why and I told him that he had no faith and had talked so about
> homeopathy.[67]

Mason replied that if he was just a "little sick" he would take it, but wanted "medicine" when he was "real sick." According to Janney, Mason was quite provoked when she told him, "If you won't take it when you are real sick, I won't give you any now."[68]

Janney advised her parents, friends, and fellow boarders on prescriptions and sometimes prepared remedies for them. Professors prescribed remedies during her own bouts of illness, and later case records show she used homeopathic remedies in practice. For Janney and the majority of homeopaths, homeopathy was a superior tool in the treatment of disease, not alternative medical knowledge.

While we can make only broad comparisons between coeducational homeopathic and regular schools, Janney's experience in BU's coeducational "experiment" was positive. Relations among female and male students and faculty appear harmonious compared with the experiences of women in regular schools. The University of Michigan in Ann Arbor was the largest, best known, and most respected of all western medical schools adopting coeducation; its decision to admit women in 1870 was hailed as the beginning of "real coeducation."[69] Yet the coeducational policy was made without the full backing of the medical faculty who petitioned for an exception, claiming subjects discussed in lectures were too delicate to be presented in mixed classes. Women students told of a difficult time. Eliza Mosher remembered that she and other women needed "strong nerves" when they attended a lecture in organic chemistry given to a mixed class of male and female students. Cat calls, a general stampede, and "lunatic" behavior by male students seemed almost to please the professor in charge, who did nothing to discourage the men.[70]

In contrast, Janney found her professors encouraging, and male students generally respectful. Her correspondence reveals only one incident when a male student answered a question "in a manner . . . insulting to the Doctor & to the whole class," inciting laughter among some. Two days later, Dean Talbot condemned the "vulgar actions" of the students, urging them to drop the medical profession if they "could not change the level of their minds."[71] According to her letters, Janney and other women students at BU found the atmosphere extremely supportive. Professors assumed women could perform as well as or better than male students, "All our Professors (or nearly all) are delighted with the success of coeducation in the college. I think they do everything to make it pleasant for us."[72]

A consistent theme in Janney's letters and a familiar one in histories of women in medicine is her desire to remain feminine, while exhibiting the necessary masculine characteristics associated with becoming a physician. Despite her nontraditional occupational choice, she held conventional views of "masculine" and "feminine" attributes. Like many women who entered the male medical world, Janney struggled to combine her identity as a lady and as a physician. Although she sought to expand and improve women's sphere by her "useful" career, her goal was to assimilate into the medical profession rather than a sisterhood of female physicians.[73] She strove to acquire such masculine strengths as emotional restraint, a steady hand while performing surgery under the eyes of faculty and students, and the fortitude to withstand disagreeable sights and smells of the dissecting room. Women who appeared too feminine in either behavior or dress risked being considered not up to the rigors of medical study and practice. And those not feminine enough confirmed the views of conservatives who warned women would be "masculinized" by the process. These tensions were the root of Janney's criticisms of many women at the school.

Janney found few women whose behavior and appearance conformed to her ideas of proper womanhood: "Some of the women are disgusting . . . if I thought it was studying medicine that made them so I would quit instantly for

I think womanliness and gentle manners are not to be lost under any circumstances."[74] Janney's overriding concern was that she not become "manly" in her
pursuit of a career dominated by men. She liked to look "graceful" and "pretty,"
and if "by submitting to a little inconvenience in long skirts I can look better, I
will submit cheerfully." She hated the "short dresses," "clumsy sacques," and
"guse-boat" like shoes and the "swinging, independent, almost defiant" manner
of many of her classmates. She was pleased at how nice she looked in the dissecting room with her "calico apron and sleeves," whereas "some of the ladies
look like frights."[75] She wrote of one woman: "The boys can't bear her. She
parts her hair on the side and is one of these ranting, masculine women . . ."[76]

Janney especially disliked Professor Mary Safford Blake who "may do an
immense amount of good but talks of 'dress reform' continually and makes herself disagreeable to many . . . she goes at the men and tells them it's their fault
that women dress as they do . . . [but] . . . it does no good to hurl it at them in
that way."[77] According to Janney, Blake looked "simply ridiculous on the ros-
trum! Her dress is so short that you can almost see the tops of her shoes and
such shoes! Run down at the heels, big enough for a woman twice her size, and
not even dusted."[78] Compounding Mary Safford Blake's faults in Janney's eyes
were her radical views on sexual relations. "Mother, I very much fear that Dr.
Blake is traveling toward that terrible free love . . . she has readings of that sort
at her house. I mean to find out positively before I make up my mind about
her."[79] But Frances Janney had already made up her mind about Mary Safford
Blake. Although Janney believed women required spunk, perseverance, and a
strong character to become doctors, the behavior and dress of Blake and several women students confirmed the worst fears of those who believed women
doctors would lose their femininity and become unsexed or manly through
exposure to the harsh realities of medical study and practice.

Janney confided her frustration to her mother: "I get so disgusted with
'Dress reform' and 'Woman's Suffrage' . . . at times, that I have almost made up
my mind never to identify myself with any society but to pursue my own independent [path]." She assured her mother that she was not going to the
extreme of "anti-dress reform" although the appearance and opinions of
women radicals made her "blood boil" sometimes.[80]

Janney's letters suggest that women students at BU expressed a more radical type of feminism than did regular women physicians in Boston. Marie
Zakrzewska, head of New England Hospital for Women and Children, regularly rejected "extremists" whose hair was cut very short or who wore reform
dress, believing they were detrimental to the highest standards of professionalism.[81] Although Janney shared those sentiments, the school's liberalism—
like that of New York Medical College and Hospital for Women—may have

increased its appeal for many women. Janney's ideas may have been more typ-ical of the second generation of women in medicine, which rejected aggres-sive tactics and the expression of radical feminism. Although we do not know the ages of the classmates who earned her disapproval, perhaps they were among the generation that pioneered the struggle for women's rights. Janney believed such women were "too asserting and too much on the offensive," and were altogether detrimental to women's professional success.[82] But despite their different concepts of feminism, the two generations represented by Jan-ney and Safford Blake shared pride in the homeopathic commitment to equal education for women. As Safford Blake noted, although BU's decision was considered an "experiment" in New England, coeducation at Hahnemann Medical College in Chicago had "long since proven a success," strengthening the connection of homeopaths with liberal reform.[83]

Expanding Educational Opportunities

With increasing numbers of both regular and homeopathic schools adopting coeducation in the last decades of the century, women's options expanded considerably. The majority of women who became homeopathic doctors did so at a time when a "regular" medical education was widely available, disprov-ing the assumption that women chose homeopathic colleges through lack of options. And while some women sought regular medical degrees because they feared their previous sectarian training would adversely affect their profes-sional lives, others who attended regular colleges switched to homeopathic schools to complete their studies. In several cases, women graduates of regular medical colleges sought post-graduate training in homeopathy.[84]

Lelia H. Powers and Annie Marchant of Maryland attended the regular Woman's Medical College of Baltimore for three years beginning in 1895. They transferred to Southern Homoeopathic Medical College in Baltimore for their final year, graduating in 1899. Mabel Sisson of Easton, New York, transferred to the homeopathic college at Boston University after one year at Woman's Medical College of Pennsylvania. Sara Allen of Philadelphia attended Woman's Medical College of Pennsylvania during her first year and transferred to Hahnemann Medical College and Hospital of Chicago for her second. During her final two years, Allen attended Hering Medical College in Chicago, a school that emphasized traditional homeopathy.[85]

We have become used to thinking about orthodox medical training as the most logical professional choice for anyone interested in a medical career in the latter part of the nineteenth century. Yet, the choice of medical college was influenced by a variety of factors. In addition to family affiliation with either regular or homeopathic medicine, women's decisions were influenced by location and climate, an institution's academic reputation, clinical opportunities, social environment, and the opinions of one's preceptor. In some cases, these factors were more determinative of one's choice than whether or not a school was regular or homeopathic.

Sometimes, attendance at a particular school reflected ambivalence or relative indifference over the directions women would take as practitioners.[86] Chicago homeopath Mary Hanks, who graduated from BU in 1897, said homeopathy had "meant very little" to her during her first year as a medical student. Describing her background as "allopathic," Hanks said her interest in homeopathy increased significantly during her second year. During that time she suffered acute tonsillitis, a recurring infection that typically lasted ten days or two weeks. With homeopathic care, however, Hanks declared she was "good as new" in three days, thereafter committing herself to the practice of homeopathy.[87]

For Julia Loos, a graduate of Woman's Medical College of Pennsylvania (WMCP) in 1894, the choice of homeopathy was clear from the beginning. Discussing the distribution of financial aid at an 1896 alumnae meeting of WMCP, Eleanor M. Hiestand-Moore, M.D., said that in one case a scholarship student had actually confided in her that she meant to practice homeopathy. Although she could not "expose" the student because of the confidential nature of the conversation, she told the young woman in plain terms that she was obtaining money under false pretenses. Although Loos was not identified by name, she was the recipient of a scholarship at WMCP early in the 1890s and the likely subject of Hiestand-Moore's consternation. Indicating that this was not the first such case, Hiestand-Moore continued: "Several times financial aid has been given to students who entered the college determined upon the practice of warming a viper."[88] After graduating from WMCP, Loos attended the Post-Graduate School of Homoeopathics in Philadelphia, becoming one of the staunchest advocates of Hahnemannian homeopathy.

Mary Ives received her doctor of medicine degree at WMCP in 1894 and attended the Philadelphia Post-Graduate School of Homoeopathics in 1895. Like Loos, Ives's choice of Philadelphia's post-graduate school with its emphasis on teaching traditional or "pure" homeopathy reflects an ideological preference. Although Ives practiced homeopathic medicine for forty-six years in Middletown, Connecticut, and was at one time president of the Connecticut Homoeopathic Medical Society, she maintained interest in her alma mater. As a member of the WMCP alumnae organization, Ives enthusiastically attended the fiftieth reunion of her graduating class in 1940.[89] Lydia Webster Stokes also attended the fiftieth reunion of her class in 1944. Graduating from WMCP in 1894, Stokes also learned homeopathy at Philadelphia's post-graduate school. Active in a number of homeopathic medical societies throughout her life and on staff at Women's Southern Homoeopathic Hospital and Dispensary from 1908 to1924, Stokes was proud of her association with WMCP. She appears among members of the alumnae association as early as 1925.[90]

In her study of women doctors in Washington, D. C., Gloria Moldow found at least seven women who switched to homeopathic medicine after graduating from Howard University. My research revealed thirty additional "converts" in various locations between 1859 and 1898—fifteen between 1890 and 1899. They became homeopathic practitioners through independent-study, apprenticeships under homeopathic physicians, or post-graduate education.[91] All were active throughout their professional lives in homeopathic medical societies, colleges, and hospitals, indicating that homeopathy did not necessarily hinder professional advancement. During the last several decades of the century, homeopathy and regular medicine gradually converged. Hostility lessened between members of both professions, and the curricula of the respective medical schools emphasized similar subjects. In many cases, lines between homeopathic and regular education and practice were quite permeable; in some circles relations among were regulars and homeopaths not as strained as the rhetoric between them suggests.

Between 1890 and 1920, changes in American medicine profoundly affected medical education and the profession itself, leading to the demise of most homeopathic colleges. But for most of this period, women homeopaths did not view themselves as disadvantaged. Active members and leaders in homeopathic professional organizations, they often developed lucrative private practices. The majority of women chose to become regular practitioners when regular medical education became more widely available; yet women homeopaths enjoyed successful medical careers and experienced a remarkable level of inclusiveness, compared to women in the medical mainstream.

For the first generation of women in medicine, a homeopathic education was not a course of least resistance. Women did not necessarily attend homeopathic medical colleges through lack of options. In their early struggles to gain admission to male-only institutions and establish separate medical colleges for women, they were similar to women in the regular profession. Yet, by the second generation of women physicians, homeopathy had developed a reputation for having a more progressive viewpoint of women in the profession than regular medicine. Much of this reputation, however, can be traced to women's own efforts. Women in the first generation of homeopathic medicine helped to forge homeopathy's identity as an enlightened, liberal-minded realm within the larger, less hospitable arena of American medicine.

Chapter 4

Adding Women to the Ranks

Nineteenth-Century Medical Societies and the Admission of Women

At THE 1869 ANNUAL MEETING of the American Institute of Homoeopathy (AIH), George W. Swazey opened discussion of "the woman question" with a formal motion. Two years earlier, a woman's application for membership had been denied by a close vote; now, he said, with no "particular lady" in the equation, his colleagues should decide the "abstract question" rather than have it "hang over us year after year." And in his opinion, the question of women's rights had nothing to do with it: "The question is whether, after having encouraged women to enter the profession, educated them, taken their money, permitted them to practice, and fraternized with them, we shall now debar them from the privilege of our larger institutions."[1] The majority of Swazey's colleagues cast their vote in favor of women's admission to the AIH the following year. Twenty-five years later, Amelia J. Burroughs of Omaha, Nebraska, reflected on those earlier years. Until the AIH membership voted to admit them, she said, women had "knocked for admittance" year after year, turning away "disappointed but not discouraged," determined to share the "benefits and power" of the national organization.[2]

Women physicians, both regulars and homeopaths, applied for admission to medical societies beginning in the 1860s—a time when regular physicians were seeking to uplift their profession. The proliferation of proprietary medical schools, designed mainly to turn a profit; the emergence of sectarian medicine; and, the demise of compulsory state licensing earlier in the century had resulted in a plethora of poorly-trained doctors and "irregular" practitioners by the last third of the century. Thus, the development of a complex range of medical societies during this time served a variety of interests.[3] Membership in a county or state medical society validated physicians' educational credentials. Membership sometimes led to staff appointments at hospitals or on public health boards, signifying one's "moral" character and good standing in the profession, and provided physicians with a list of approved colleagues for consultations or referrals. Membership was important to full participation in both the homeopathic and regular medical professions, and women actively sought admission throughout the last decades of the nineteenth century.[4]

Women's struggle for inclusion in male regular medical societies has been well documented by historians.[5] In many instances, women homeopaths faced similar opposition. But unlike women regulars, who often established separate medical societies as an indirect route to professional assimilation, women were active participants in homeopathic organizations. They expressed opinions, demonstrated leadership abilities, and influenced the directions of these organizations, elevating women's status within the profession. The inclusion and collegiality women experienced in homeopathic medical societies as well as their early acceptance by particular homeopathic medical societies and colleges, suggests that male homeopathic physicians made a ideological commitment to women's equal opportunity. Perhaps the ideological and numerical minority status of homeopaths made them more sensitive to the struggles of other marginal groups. However, the apparent liberality of homeopaths also served the needs of the profession.

Comparing controversies over admitting women to the American Medical Association, the American Institute of Homoeopathy, and regular and homeopathic medical societies in Pennsylvania and Massachusetts, reveals that—more than reform ideology—competitive and antagonistic relations between homeopaths and regulars as well as divisiveness within the homeopathic profession, affected debates and decisions on women's admission. Professional opportunities for women in both schools of medicine were shaped by interprofessional competition and accommodation, which, in turn, were greatly influenced by the intersection of gender and sectarianism. Directly and indirectly homeopathy played an essential role in recasting the physician from a medically educated male to a practitioner of either sex, shifting debates away from gender toward proper education and practice.

Opening Doors

By turn of the century, women homeopaths had been active in homeopathic medical societies for over a quarter century. After the doors to the AIH were

opened to them in 1871, women became active participants in the organization, presenting papers and case reports at annual meetings, chairing committees, and contributing to decisions on institutional policy. By 1904, seven
women had served as vice presidents of the AIH. Records of the International
Hahnemannian Association (IHA) show a similar level of participation by
women. Although not among the organization's fifty-nine founders, women
were actively involved in the organization within a decade. The IHA held
annual meetings in different cities across the United States, spawning numerous local Hahnemannian organizations. By 1898, women numbered fifteen
out of one hundred and six active and associate members. Between 1896 to
1915, women chaired the board of censors and bureau sections; seven were
elected vice presidents, and two served additional terms. Both the AIH and
IHA drew women members primarily from Massachusetts, New York, Illinois,
Pennsylvania, Michigan, and California.[6]

Sometimes attendance at meetings of regional homeopathic societies
exceeded the annual conventions of the two national groups. Closer to home,
these meetings lacked the geographic divisiveness sometimes evident at the
national gatherings. Women assumed early and active leadership roles. From
the 1870s to the early 1900s, the following regional medical societies elected
women to their executive boards: Northwestern Pennsylvania Homoeopathic
Medical Society, Homoeopathic Medical Society of Southwest Michigan,
Homoeopathic Medical Society of Northern Pennsylvania, and Western
Massachusetts Homoeopathic Medical Society. In 1896, Lizzie Gray Gutherz
of Kentucky became president of the Southern Homoeopathic Medical Association, the second largest homeopathic society in the country.[7]

This pattern prevailed in state, county, and city homeopathic societies.
As early as 1874, Clara Yeomans of Iowa became the first woman vice president of a state society. Throughout the latter decades of the nineteenth century, nine state organizations elected women to their executive boards,
including Kansas, Illinois, Florida, Nebraska, California, Colorado, Pennsylvania, New Jersey, and Connecticut. And in 1900, Adelaide Lambert of Connecticut became the first president of a state homeopathic organization.[8] The
Homoeopathic Medical Society of Chicago, one of the most prestigious
county societies, elected Mary Elizabeth Hanks president in 1904. Two years
later she became president of the Homoeopathic Medical Society of the state
of Illinois, one of the largest state organizations.[9] Chicago women were particularly active in this organization.

Ten years after the AIH voted to admit women, however, some male colleagues complained that women took little part in enlarging the homeopathic
materia medica. They hoped that after becoming members, women would add

to the homeopathic materia medica by conducting provings, enlarging the pharmacoepia with drugs specifically tested on women. One physician lamented: "their contributions to the materia medica and therapeutics have been meagre in the extreme." Another suggested that women-only medical societies might provide the best context for such work, that perhaps women had collected many facts, but were too modest to present them in a mixed group.[10]

However, countless examples contradict the notion of women's shyness at professional meetings, revealing that women were neither more nor less productive than male colleagues in drug testing. As more women became members, they presented many provings and cases for discussion to the membership of the AIH. And at least one women's organization had a clearly defined scientific objective. In 1893, at the World Homoeopathic Congress held in conjunction with Chicago's Columbian Exposition, women founded the International Women Provers Union, making a formal effort to expand the homeopathic pharmacopea with drugs effective in treating women's illnesses. Although originally organized with a vice president in each state to supervise the work of women provers, the organization seems to have consisted of several regional groups that presented their findings to the AIH. Millie Chapman, a driving force behind women's drug proving, was vice president and then president of the new organization, in addition to her appointment within the AIH as head of the Committee on Drug Proving (1895).[11]

Although women homeopaths established separate societies, they did not do so nearly as frequently as women regular physicians.[12] I located only four such organizations: the Women's Homoeopathic Medical Association of Chicago (1879); the Women's Homoeopathic Medical Club of Allegheny County, Pennsylvania (established around 1900); the Women's Homoeopathic Medical Association of Pittsburgh, Pennsylvania (1900); and the Women's Medical Club of Philadelphia (1883). The Chicago association maintained its separate existence from 1879 to 1886 when it joined with other Chicago groups to establish the Protective Agency for Women and Children—later known as Legal Aid.[13] In 1925 the Pittsburgh association celebrated its twenty-fifth anniversary and honored its first president, Millie J. Chapman, one of Pittsburgh's first female doctors. An ardent champion of women's rights, and one of homeopathy's most active promoters, Chapman joined and led several professional organizations at the state and national levels. Though a small organization, the Pittsburgh society comprised some of Pennsylvania's leading women physicians—Julia Loos, Anna Johnston, Ella D. Goff, and Anna Varner—all active in other homeopathic societies.[14] Harriet J. Sartain, the organization's first president, retained the office for many years, even after her retirement from active practice.[15] Besides its social and educational functions, the Women's Homoeopathic Medical Club of Philadelphia had a clearly identified political agenda. Chafing under the male-only policy of Hahnemann Medical College, members worked in vain to change its admissions policy which excluded women.

Historians have argued that within regular medicine, women's medical societies developed not from women's exclusion from regular medical organizations, but in communities accepting of women physicians. Societies often encouraged women to join, invited them to give papers and to hold office, and appointed them as delegates to annual conventions of other societies. Ellen More suggests that while women's medical societies were instruments of professional integration and legitimization, they fused the professional values of medicine with Victorian values of "female benevolence, social reform, and civic activism"—elements of social feminism that initially attracted many women to the profession.[16]

As regular medical associations opened their doors to women, however, many chose not to participate actively. One historian suggests that minority status may have led to feelings of isolation, causing women not to take active roles.[17] The ratios of women to men in the following state societies support this possibility: Connecticut, 8:500 (1982), Minnesota, 9:380 (1886), Iowa, 21:760 (1903), and New York, 4:600 (1899).[18] Women homeopaths were also a small minority in homeopathic organizations. Yet, judging from their high level of involvement in a variety of formerly male-only medical societies and the establishment of very few separate organizations, women homeopaths preferred a more direct method of integration into their profession. As the following comparison of women in Pennsylvania shows, they were extremely involved in the state homeopathic society.

Women Physicians in Pennsylvania

For nineteen years between 1881 and 1900, women were members of the Board of Censors of the Homoeopathic Medical Society of the State of Pennsylvania. Beginning in 1885, women chaired and became members of the individual bureaus of gynecology, paedology (children's health), obstetrics, clinical medicine, and sanitary science.[19] At yearly meetings, at least two or three women presented papers on subjects such as tonsillitis, poliomyelitis, menopause, and the efficacy of homeopathic remedies in pelvic disease and fibroid tumors. In 1891, Millie Chapman became second vice president of the state society, and a woman was appointed delegate from the Pennsylvania society to the Southern Homoeopathic Medical Association. From 1892 to 1894, women served as first and second vice presidents, and in 1900, Ella Goff became treasurer, a position she held for two years. Women frequently presented papers and cases at annual meetings, and participated actively in professional discussions.[20]

In sharp contrast, proceedings of the regular medical society of Pennsylvania reveal no such participation by women. None served on the executive board during this period, nor were they censors or members of specialty committees. Although members presented six papers, the same woman physician wrote four of them.[21] In 1897, approximately 14 percent of Philadelphia's regular women physicians belonged to the AMA, 41 percent of the city's women homeopaths belonged to the AIH. A slightly higher percentage of women regulars belonged to state and county societies (25 percent), while the same percentage of homeopaths (41 percent) belonged to their state and local societies.[22]

In 1897 the Homoeopathic Medical Society of the State of Pennsylvania listed 234 members; only eleven were women. Yet, at the annual meeting, attended by approximately half the entire membership, nine women were present with eight serving on specialty bureaus. In contrast, women regulars had the opportunity of support from a larger number of female colleagues at meetings. In 1895, the regular society of Pennsylvania listed 1,590 members, fifty of whom were women. The Philadelphia county society showed twenty-three women out of 648 members, yet their level of participation was lower than the smaller number of women homeopaths in their county and state organizations.

Some historians have argued that the problem for women in medical societies toward the end of the century was not exclusion, but their own rejection of a professional ethos defined by competitive values and aggressive individualism. Women's values of cooperation and mutual support often conflicted with the "narrow professionalism and crass materialism" they found characteristic of male colleagues.[23] The ideals of social feminism—the health of women and children, public health, and social hygiene—were gradually subsumed by the rising technical and scientific aspects of medicine beginning in the last decade of the century. Reductionist tendencies influenced by the growing reliance on laboratory evidence and the identification of specific diseases narrowed the clinical view, diminishing the importance of patients' habits, idiosyncrasies, family history, character, work, and worries. By the time women were admitted to most medical societies, a new professional ethos shaped by the "scientific objectivity" of medicine as an applied science diverged from an earlier, more holistic model of medical practice.[24] And as Ellen More argues, when collegial professionalism began to diverge from the broad-based civic and social concerns of an earlier generation of physicians, women's medical societies were a means of prolonging their compatibility.[25]

Although homeopaths were also influenced by the new directions in medicine, perhaps homeopathic societies were governed by a less technocratic ethos, one more compatible with women's values and ideals. Perhaps the minority status of male homeopaths made them more sensitive to women's struggle for recognition and inclusion, enhancing collegiality within organizations. The definition of homeopaths by regulars as the "other" may have encouraged cohesiveness among homeopathic men and women. Medical societies not only promoted continuing education but also engaged physicians in the progress of the profession. For women in the homeopathic profession, integration rather than separation was a more effective strategy of assimilation, a fact that male homeopaths often pointed to as evidence of their progressiveness on the "woman question." Within both schools of medicine, however, women's professional opportunities as well as decisions to admit women to medical societies were influenced by local political, socioeconomic, and professional factors intertwined with gender and sectarianism.

Comparing Women's Admission to the AIH and AMA

When members of the American Institute of Homoeopathy cast their votes in favor of women's admission in 1869, they did so amidst discussions of why their school of medicine should lead the way in recognizing women's rightful place in the medical profession. They mentioned fairness, the benefits of being considered more socially progressive than regular physicians, as well as the need to serve homeopathy's largest constituency. But discussions also reveal intraprofessional tensions over what constituted proper homeopathic practice.

As Regina Morantz-Sanchez has shown, the justification for women as physicians often rested upon their presumed moral superiority and the womanly virtues of patience, tenderness, and sensitivity.[26] While this was also true in homeopathy, the profession's leaders used another, more compelling argument to convince reluctant colleagues that women should be welcomed as full participants in the profession. They were needed as testers or "provers" of drugs for the homeopathic materia medica.

Clearly, homeopathic physicians considered, homeopathic therapeutics especially effective for women's and children's diseases. Contemporary estimates were that women comprised two-thirds of all patients, and those in the profession believed their "conversion" was critical to the survival and growth of homeopathy. The treatment of women's diseases, however, required remedies "proved" on healthy women. Conducting such provings was the work of physicians under direction of the AIH, with organizational help provided by local medical societies. However, most physicians up to this time had been men; and by 1870, AIH leaders showed great concern for more and better testing of drugs for women's diseases.[27] Carroll Dunham reminded his colleagues of the importance of a woman's contributions to the improvement of the materia medica, "with her different equilibrium of intellect and physique, with her special and distinctive tests of drugs."[28] If remedies could be made more effective, perhaps homeopaths would be less inclined to stray from traditional or orthodox homeopathic practices by prescribing multiple remedies and doses, or turning to nonhomeopathic therapeutics. Leaders hoped that more effective remedies would quell the escalating divisiveness among homeopaths over what constituted proper homeopathic prescribing. Also, more control and precision in the testing of drugs would approximate new methods of investigation being developed within modern laboratory medicine. But Dunham warned it was unlikely women physicians would be convinced to take up the work of provings, ". . . unless they were recognized and received by us as fellow workers on an equal footing in every respect."[29] Dr. David Thayer echoed these pleas. Thayer, who as a member of the Massachusetts legislature, was instrumental in securing a charter for the homeopathic medical school at Boston University, and argued the folly of only involving "one-half the brains of the race" in improving the "indispensable science" of homeopathy. "Science," said Thayer, "should accept help from every quarter."[30]

Heightened concern over improving the materia medica at this particular time may be seen as an effort by the AIH to get its house in order. When members voted to admit women, they did so amidst calls for liberty of medical opinion and arguments over whether to exclude certain physicians based on their "unhomeopathic" ideas or practices. The controversies were stimulated in large part by the changing ideals of medical science in the last third of the nineteenth century. Increasing numbers of regular practitioners believed that legitimate physicians would be identified by their scientific knowledge rather than by their adherence to therapeutic principles, codes of conduct, or medical systems. Beginning in the 1870s, debates in several regular medical societies questioned the rationale behind the code of ethics of the AMA, prohibiting consultation with homeopaths. As one professor told his students in 1872: "Modern science is indifferent to Hippocrates and Hahnemann. If their theories will not bear the bright light of the present, let them wander back into the darkness of the past to which they belong. . . . The therapeutics of today reject dogmas, and the therapeutics of the future will accept nothing that can not be demonstrated by the tests of science."[31]

The majority of homeopaths regarded the liberalizing tendencies among regulars and the potential of laboratory science to support and confirm homeopathic principles as evidence of progress. The smaller but influential group of

Hahnemannians viewed the liberal stirrings as a threat to homeopathy as a separate medical system, believing that homeopathic principles were wholly incompatible with those of regular medicine. Hahnemannians insisted the views and practices of their more liberal colleagues in the AIH violated the only reliable guide to therapeutics, Samuel Hahnemann's *Organon.* They considered themselves the only legitimate voices of pure homeopathy, proclaiming most homeopaths "mongrels" and an even greater danger to their profession than allopaths.[32]

In 1869, when AIH members voted that the organization should be open to all who expressed an interest in learning and practicing homeopathy, despite their nonhomeopathic practices, Hahnemannians reacted with "regret and gloomy forebodings."[33] Professional tolerance of colleagues whose practices did not fully conform to Hahnemann's teachings gave way to vituperative criticism, causing one physician to note: "In the hour of our bondage, when proscription stared us in the face, we were a band of brothers, . . . but now prosperity makes us more vicious, and 'rule or ruin' seems to be more and more the fundamental idea of a professional life."[34] And in arguments over whom should be considered a homeopathic physician, loyalty to either progressive or traditional homeopathic ideology ranked above gender as an area of professional concern to male homeopaths.

When leading homeopaths insisted that female physicians were critical to the continuance and expansion of homeopathic science, they added a compelling argument for women's admission to national and local homeopathic societies. The emphasis on women's role as provers at this late date, however, reflects the anxieties of those physicians who were interested in modernizing homeopathy in accordance with new scientific ideals by updating and improving the homeopathic materia medica. As one physician noted, the decision to admit them [women] stemmed not so much from gallantry or justice but from the ". . . highest regards to the interests of the Institute."[35]

Unlike homeopathy, orthodox medicine lacked a specific framework wherein women physicians made unique contributions to the science of their profession—although in the practice of medicine they were presumed morally superior, patient, tender, and sensitive. Nor were women regular physicians considered useful allies in internecine struggles. Debates over women's admission during the 1871 AMA convention occasioned exuberant applause for arguments on both sides. The metaphorical language showed the tremendous pressures felt by physicians over the inevitability of women in the profession and the dangers of not yielding. One speaker warned, "the longer you oppose resistance to this current, the stronger it becomes by opposing it . . . We shall add the force of Niagara to the current that is coming down upon us . . ." He insisted opponents of women's admission weakened the bonds connecting them with many of the "brightest luminaries" within medicine such as Alfred Stillé, president of the AMA, and others associated with female institutions. Dr. Harding warned members that the regular profession should find a place for women in its institutions, or they would be driven into "that *ism* or that *pathy* and the best interests of the science of medicine will be injured."[36]

Although there was de facto acceptance of women beginning in 1876, when Dr. Sarah Hackett Stevenson was seated as a delegate from Chicago, the AMA did not change its bylaws regarding the admission of women until 1915.[37] In contrast, during the year Stevenson took her seat as a delegate, the American Institute of Homoeopathy counted twenty-seven women members with full voting rights and privileges. And by that time, ten women had been elected to serve as vice presidents and one as secretary to that organization.

Local Medical Societies

While national medical societies argued the abstract question of women's admission, local organizations of physicians often had "particular ladies" in mind as they debated the issue. In some cases, the issue was decided with little or no polemics, based on the reputation of a particular applicant. In 1866, Philadelphia homeopath Harriet Judd Sartain was one of fifty-eight founding members of the Philadelphia County Homoeopathic Society. In 1872, she was the first woman admitted to the Homoeopathic Medical Society of the State of Pennsylvania.[38] When Sartain gained membership in Pennsylvania's professional homeopathic organizations, she had one of the most successful medical practices in Philadelphia, irrespective of sex.[39] She was not only a prominent homeopathic physician but also a member of one of the city's most socially elite families through her marriage to Samuel Sartain, son of celebrated Philadelphia engraver John Sartain. She counted among her friends leading male physicians of both schools of medicine, including homeopaths William B. Van Lennep and Pemberton Dudley, both on the faculty of Hahnemann Medical College, as well as notable regulars such as D. Hayes Agnew and S. Weir Mitchell.[40] Perhaps Sartain's elevated social position and prestigious professional associations encouraged consensus; no debates or discussion of "the woman question" took place in either the county or the state homeopathic society. Upon admitting women, both organizations encouraged their active participation.

But women's ready acceptance into the county and state homeopathic societies of Philadelphia and Pennsylvania also may have been influenced by a lack of potential applicants. Directories show only six women homeopaths in Philadelphia in 1870 and only thirteen throughout the state.[41] Because women were prohibited from matriculating at Hahnemann Medical College in Philadelphia—the largest homeopathic medical school in the country— the vast majority of homeopaths in Pennsylvania were male. Thus, while Pennsylvania's male homeopaths appeared liberal due to the lack of contentious debates over women's admission as well as the election of women to important roles within homeopathic societies, their ideological commitment to women's rights was sometimes subsumed by the proprietary interests of homeopathic institutions.

Within regular medical societies, debates over the admission of women intertwined with the American Medical Association's opposition to homeopathy. As part of its program to set national standards, the AMA formulated the consultation clause of the code of ethics (1847), regulating professional relations between orthodox and other medical systems, especially homeopathy. In 1855, member societies were required to adopt the code; and after the Civil War, when the popularity of homeopathy increased significantly, the AMA required its member societies to expel "irregular" members from its affiliated societies.[42] Events in Pennsylvania were particularly striking illustrations of these forces.

Pennsylvania

Philadelphia was a major center for every segment of medical education: regular and homeopathic, single-sex and coed. The presence of Hahnemann Medical College, Woman's Medical College of Pennsylvania, and the eclectic Penn Medical University resulted in large numbers of homeopaths and women physicians remaining in the area to establish medical practices.[43] In 1859, the Medical Society of Pennsylvania decided upon a broad interpretation of the consultation clause, insisting that because many women physicians graduated from sectarian institutions, and because some faculty members of regular female medical colleges were "irregular," women's medical education was tainted by sectarian influences. The laws of the state society, they said, required expulsion of doctors who consulted with female physicians.

Members of the Montgomery county society, a small organization of rural practitioners, found the argument of the Philadelphia physicians specious, using it to further the interests of men waging a war against female physicians. At a meeting of the state medical society in 1860, Hiram Corson, whose niece Sarah Adamson Dolley graduated from medical school in 1851, presented a resolution on behalf of the Montgomery Medical Society to test the sincerity of Philadelphia physicians.[44] The resolution called for admission into medical societies of women instructed by "well-qualified and legitimate teachers," conforming to the medical code established by the AMA. This resolution failed, with the Philadelphia county society spearheading its defeat at the state level.[45]

Taken to its logical conclusion, the state society's rule prohibited any physician from consulting male physicians on the faculty of women's medical colleges, or who served as consultants in hospitals run by women physicians. This posed a problem, since many of the state's most prominent physicians were consultants for female-run institutions. For example, when Dr. Ann Preston, former dean of the Woman's Medical College of Pennsylvania, headed the medical staff of Woman's Hospital in Philadelphia, Alfred Stillé, president of the AMA, and other notables such as John Forsyth Meigs and S. Weir Mitchell were consulting physicians to the hospital.[46] Many of these physicians also belonged to the College of Physicians of Philadelphia, a medical organization whose Fellows were among the most elite practitioners and educators in the state. Not a representative organization of the state society, and therefore not subject to its rules, the College of Physicians freely consulted with women physicians and their institutions, supporting women's full inclusion in the profession through membership in *other* medical societies. Fellows of the college had little sympathy for their Pennsylvania colleagues, considering the dilemma of the county and state societies one of their own making.[47]

Impatient with the controversy generated by the Philadelphia physicians, the AMA refused to provide the clarification sought by the county organization. Although the debate over women's admission flared within the AMA as well, the "gentlemen" in Philadelphia and Pennsylvania were left to "manage their own quarrels." The AMA did not agree (or disagree) with the argument that women, by virtue of their visible or invisible ties to sectarian medicine, should be excluded from medical societies under the consultation clause of the code of ethics.[48]

Alongside the obvious issues of gender and sectarianism in these debates, lay equally divisive elements of economics and class. Competition was vigorous for a regular, nonelite male physician trying to make a living in and around Philadelphia. In 1870, only New York City exceeded Philadelphia's physician population.[49] Members of the prestigious College of Physicians could afford their liberal stance on the issue of consulting with women. Physicians such as S. Weir Mitchell, Walter Atlee, and Alfred Stillé, the latter two former presidents of the AMA, did not fear for the economic viability of their medical practices nor their social and professional status in Philadelphia. For those less well situated, the county and state interpretation of the consultation clause offered some protection for medical practices.

But how do we explain the minority position of professionally secure members of the College of Physicians who opposed any association with women physicians? Rejecting the liberal views of many of their colleagues, several voted to support members of the Philadelphia county society in their opposition to women's admission. Economic self-interest does not explain the actions of D. Hayes Agnew, distinguished surgeon of the University of Pennsylvania and Pennsylvania Hospital, who resigned in 1869 when hospital managers decided to admit women physicians to the clinics. Squier Littell, Agnew's colleague in the College of Physicians, presented a resolution condemning the managers for their usurpation of the physicians' authority. When a majority of members failed to vote for the resolution, Agnew resigned his position at the hospital "rather than submit to such dictation." Littell commended him for vindicating his own "dignity and independence."[50] For Agnew, the challenge to his growing authority, not his financial status, explains his adverse reaction to women in clinics.

Concern for economics, status, and authority explains the opposition to women's membership by many physicians in Philadelphia. Rural physicians, however, generally favored women's inclusion in professional organizations—perhaps because they did not face the same kinds of competition. According to the U.S. Census of 1870, of the thirty-nine women physicians practicing in the state of Pennsylvania, twenty-six were located in Philadelphia.[51] One hundred and thirty-four male homeopaths practiced in Philadelphia, whereas only sixty were located in rural areas and small towns.[52] The results of an 1867 vote by delegates to the Pennsylvania state medical society reveal that seven out of nine county societies favored consultation with "properly educated women" and their admission into the ranks of the profession—but the measure failed to pass. The Lancaster county medical society "was instructed [by the Philadelphia county society] to vote unanimously against this and all resolutions recognizing women as members of the medical profession."[53] With opposition from the more numerous delegates of the Philadelphia and Lancaster societies, urban physicians were able to out vote their rural colleagues.

At yearly meetings throughout the 1860s, the state society debated the issue, and each year voted down the resolution favoring women's admission proposed by the Montgomery society. In 1871, the state organization finally voted to open its doors to women; yet, six years passed before Melissa A. Bradley of Wilkes-Barre and Mary Alice Swazye of Pottsville became the first female members.[54] But unlike the state homeopathic society, no women were elected to the executive board throughout the nineteenth century, nor were they appointed to special committees.[55] In 1874, the Philadelphia county society revised its bylaws, omitting all references to the subject of women's admission. Not until 1888, after rejecting several nominees, did the society accept its first woman member.[56]

Massachusetts

If the AMA's consultation clause sparked debates involving gender and sectarianism in Pennsylvania, in Massachusetts it was a virtual lightning rod for controversy. In 1853 Nancy Talbot Clark, a graduate of Western Reserve Medical College of Cleveland, and sister of Boston's most prominent homeopath, Israel Talbot, sought validation of her medical credentials—not membership—from the regular Massachusetts Medical Society.[57] Her request was denied, but her petition triggered two decades of debates over women's physiological and educational "suitability" to practice medicine. By the 1870s, these discussions focused on women's "inherent tendencies" toward sectarianism, revealing the social and professional pressures felt by regular physicians in Boston, where the popularity of both homeopathy and women physicians were on the rise.

Connections between gender and sectarianism were reinforced by specific events in Boston, particularly the expulsion of homeopaths from the Massachusetts Medical Society and the founding of the homeopathic coeducational medical school at Boston University. Thus, the decision of the Massachusetts Homoeopathic Medical Society to elect its first female members was influenced by a variety of factors, including the backing of influential liberal physicians such as Israel Talbot and David Thayer; public pressure on homeopaths to admit women to their college; and the continuing need of homeopathic institutions for fund-raising support by Massachusetts women. And, in the aftermath of their ignominious ousting from the regular medical society of Massachusetts, homeopaths capitalized on assumptions of their own comparative liberality. In April 1874, the Massachusetts Homoeopathic Medical Society held its first meeting in the halls of the new college. Without discussion or one dissenting vote, four women homeopathic physicians, including two faculty members, were voted into membership.[58]

When the committee studying women's admission to the regular Massachusetts Medical Society reported to that organization in 1875, events of the past few years had clearly influenced the thinking of its members. Samuel Fisk argued that women's attraction to sectarian medicine presented a risk to the society. "Now we all know how easily women are led by their fancies. Today the greater part of all quackery is supported by them. I don't believe that it would be possible to keep them within the rules of the Society."[59] Fisk felt sure that censorship and expulsion of women would be inevitable because of their supposed attraction to irregular medicine. His concern had some foundation, as evidenced by the number of women in Boston's city directory listed as homeopaths, midwives, electricians, clairvoyants, eclectics, specialists in cancer and botanical cures, and baunscheidtist therapy.[60] Indeed, many first-generation women physicians, prohibited from matriculating at regular medical colleges, had received their degrees from irregular institutions.[61] By 1875, fifty-three women were enrolled in the homeopathic Boston University School of Medicine. Fisk warned fellow physicians that if women became members, and one needed to be expelled, the "expulsion of a few homeopaths would be a slight affair in comparison," and he doubted that the members would be able to "bear with composure" the gibes and abuse from the public press for "our alleged bigotry and intolerance."[62]

On the other hand, those favoring the admission of women with regular medical degrees used the connection between women and sectarianism as an argument for strengthening the professional standing of properly educated physicians. Henry Ingersoll Bowditch, a consulting physician to the New England Hospital for Women and Children, believed women were often driven into sectarian medicine. He argued that the society should offer women a route to full participation in the regular profession, thereby reducing the number of sectarians, decreasing the income of their colleges, and eroding public support. In 1884 when members finally changed the organization's bylaws to admit qualified women, Bowditch's argument carried more meaning. By that time, 121 women had graduated from Boston's homeopathic medical school, and women homeopaths practicing in Boston outnumbered regular women practitioners almost two to one.[63] For those who supported women's admission, membership would separate the wheat from the chaff. Concerned that hundreds of "ill educated" women were practicing within the state of Massachusetts and that Boston University was adding annually to that number, he called upon his fellow physicians to determine the "worthiness" of individual women physicians.[64]

Women in Boston urged physicians to do just that. Three hundred and fifty women expressed their desire for competent women practitioners by presenting a petition to the regular society in 1882; by 1883, a poll of the entire membership of the Massachusetts Medical Society showed a large majority in favor of women's admission. In addition, leading citizens called for the enactment of broadly defined medical licensing laws. Boston members of the regular society opposed such legislation, fearing they would have to serve on boards alongside eclectics and homeopaths; therefore, the fair treatment of women applicants was incumbent upon the society if it wished to remain the sole arbiter of physicians' qualifications to practice medicine. In September

1884, Emma Call, a regular physician on the staff of New England Hospital, became the first female member of the Massachusetts Medical Society.[65]

Although women were not "driven" into homeopathy through lack of options, conflicts between homeopaths and regulars, as well as between traditional and progressive homeopaths, resulted in a favorable climate for women homeopathic practitioners. Through interprofessional competition and accommodation, women homeopaths facilitated women's admission to regular medical societies. Thus, homeopathy played a critical role in reconstructing the definition of physician to include properly educated practitioners of either sex.

Arguments connecting gender to sectarianism were useful for nonelite, urban practitioners eager to protect their practices from the competition of women and successful physicians. They were also used by some elite physicians in attempts to maintain the prerogatives of traditional male medical authority. And while homeopathy's stated commitment to women, both as patients and as physicians, was partly driven by the liberal and egalitarian impulses of its leaders, it was also furthered by the practical interests of the profession. For the majority of homeopathic and regular physicians alike, votes to admit women to medical societies reflected changing attitudes about women—but even more, they indicated the pragmatic desire of these physicians to serve their own best interests.

| "Women's Diseases" and |
| Homeopathic Patients, |
| Chapter 5 | 1850–1900 |

In 1869 A PATIENT suffering from "disturbed" menstrual functions, including pain in the back, dysmenorrhea, leukorrhea, and vaginismus, sought the advice of Saint Louis, Missouri, physician Thomas Griswold Comstock. The woman had previously been under the care of a homeopath who, Comstock said, made no local examination of her case (meaning vaginal exam), "but studied her subjective symptoms night and day for months." For one year the woman received various high-potency remedies including sulfur, nux vomica (poison-nut), ignatia (Saint Ignatius bean), platina (the metal), aloes (socotrine aloes), belladonna (deadly nightshade), and silicea (pure flint). Her condition steadily worsened. After acquiring her case, Comstock "demanded at once a vaginal examination." The patient at first refused being "a strong-minded woman, and opposed to the speculum."[1]

Dr. Comstock finally convinced his patient to undergo a digital examination, and administered chloroform because of the great pain she experienced. He introduced a uterine probe or "sound" and met with an obstruction in the cavity of the uterus, implying a retroflexion of the uterus as well as a tumor. He tried without success to reposition the uterus, but the woman's painful swelling and inflammation prevented more aggressive therapy at this time, so he sent her home, "ordered her to take a vaginal douche of hot water once daily, and a hip-bath of warm water, every second night," and prescribed a dose of belladonna, three times a day.[2]

After two weeks, Comstock examined the woman again, giving her a few inhalations of sulfuric ether instead of chloroform. "Ordering" his patient in the knee and elbow position, he introduced the sound, inserted his left index finger into her rectum, pressed the tumor upwards and forwards and at the same time turned the uterine sound succeeding "perfectly in elevating the tumour and replacing the uterus." Not surprisingly, the patient fainted after the operation, but according to Dr. Comstock, she soon recovered. "I kept her on her back for a week, and introduced the sound several times to assure myself that the retroflexion had not returned." He prescribed a daily vaginal douche of a gallon of hot water under hydrostatic pressure "as hot as she could bear." After restoring the retroflexed womb, Comstock chose a Hodge closed-lever pessary and an abdominal supporter to maintain the proper position of the uterus and strengthen the "lax abdominal walls."[3]

Although perhaps shocking, the treatments and procedures Comstock described in 1869 were commonly used by physicians in treating menstrual irregularities supposedly caused by uterine displacements. More surprising, however, is that Comstock himself was a homeopath. Already a trained physician when he entered the Homoeopathic Medical College of Pennsylvania around 1852, Comstock was similar to many converts from the "old school," who "gladly accepted procedures that appeared worthwhile from either school of medicine.

Contrary to present-day assumptions that homeopaths offered decidedly different alternatives to the therapeutics of regular physicians, homeopathic obstetricians and gynecologists differed from regulars more in theory than in practice. Although homeopaths faulted regular physicians for improper uterine therapeutics and accused them of contributing to rather than meliorating the sufferings of women, homeopathic practitioners often employed the very same practices, sharing the view of their regular colleagues that women's sexual organs were particularly prone to pathology and derangement. Unlike hydropaths who considered female physiological processes such as menstruation and menopause natural and nonpathological, homeopaths and regulars alike believed that women were particularly vulnerable to disequilibrium during these especially critical periods, which required medical vigilance.[4] Indeed, women's vulnerability provided homeopaths with a special arena for the promotion of homeopathic remedies as an alternative.

Women's patronage was critical to a physician's ability to make a living in areas where a plentiful supply of regular and "irregular" doctors meant stiff competition for paying patients. Contemporaries estimated women comprised two-thirds of all homeopathic patients—roughly similar to the composition of patients of regular doctors.[5] Yet we know comparatively little about women's experiences of homeopathic care during the second half of the century. What difference did it make to women whether one's physician was a regular or a homeopath? Did they have definite expectations of homeopathic treatment? And in what ways did women themselves influence medical procedures and practices?

"The Great Mother of Us All"

In the middle of the nineteenth century, homeopaths were extraordinarily optimistic about the mild, mysterious power of homeopathic remedies to create a healthy, vigorous new race. Like regular physicians, they subscribed to the view that constitutional tendencies were inherited, and that individuals could alter these over time through proper attention to the laws of nature.[6] But according to homeopaths, the "baneful practices of allopathic medicine," transmitted to the infant generation, would result in a weak and diminished race of people through the common use of venesection, forceps, drugs such as opium or laudanum, cathartics, and ergot in the treatment of parturient women. They claimed a woman under the care of a homeopathic physician from her birth would not only be spared most illnesses and derangement of internal organs, but also would transmit an improved constitution to her offspring.[7]

Calling the therapeutics of regular physicians in the treatment of women's diseases the "greatest medical scandal of the age," homeopaths believed their system would give the "death blow" to the regulars' "disgusting management of uterine and vaginal disease."[8] Accusing regular physicians of maltreating women, homeopaths blamed "women's diseases" on illness-producing drugs, procedures designed to cure them, and the improper management of parturition leading to prolapsed uteri, vesico-vaginal and recto-vaginal fistulas, perineal tears, and undefined "womb trouble."[9] Popular home-health manuals and pamphlets authored by homeopathic physicians warned of the dangers of conventional treatment, promising women a safer and more comfortable route to health through homeopathy, influencing women's expectations for significantly different, less interventionist, homeopathic care.

From the plethora of nineteenth-century literature on so-called "women's diseases," one is tempted to call it "The Uterine Century." Considered the core of the female body, an organ of significant power, the uterus was central to the function of procreation and, by extension, to the family and society as a whole. In the words of one medical student, the womb is "the great mother of us all."[10] The physician's role was to define women's duties in regard to the healthy functioning of her uterus and sexual organs, discover and diagnose evidence of malfunction, minister to an extraordinary variety of perceived derangement or displacements, and explain the causes and effects of disease.

Victorian women's duties included, not only a properly-ordered domestic sphere, but also a properly-positioned internal organization.[11]

Physicians believed the proper placement, functioning, and health of the uterus was not only central to an individual woman's ability to bear children but also, according to the theory of reflex irritation, critical to the physical, psychological, and moral functioning of the whole woman. Medical theory postulated that the uterus and ovaries were connected by sympathetic and sacral nerves to all other organs, and any disruptions in normal functioning could have wide-ranging pathological effects.[12] Combined with the belief that the human body possessed a finite amount of nerve force, and that this store of energy was smaller in females than in males, these assumptions formed the basis of an ideological system often used by conservatives to circumscribe women's role in society.

Menstruation functioned as a barometer allowing for a measurable, monthly indication of a woman's health and, by implication, her adherence to approved laws of health and society. Male homeopaths and regulars alike agreed on its importance as an indicator of good health as well as its debilitating potential. The definition of "normal" menstruation was an observable and measurable indication that women were adhering to acceptable medical and social prescriptions of dress, behavior, diet, and education. Physicians emphasized the importance of deviations in quantity, timing, and appropriate age of menstruation and their effect on the general health of females, believing that almost every action or thought of the young girl affected her future procreative abilities.[13] Women homeopaths did not challenge the notion that women were particularly prone to uterine disease resulting from their own ignorance or carelessness in regard to the laws of health. Narrowly defined physiological norms, women's role in contributing to many of their own problems, and the physician's importance as instructor and educator were consistent themes throughout the nineteenth century among both regular and homeopath physicians.

At mid-century, homeopathic treatment of menstrual irregularities consisted primarily of homeopathic remedies accompanied by hygenic measures. For example, in the case of "young ladies" of "mild character" whose menses were delayed, recommended treatment included an easily-digestible diet; avoidance of spicy foods and stimulants such as tea and coffee; and homeopathic remedies chosen according to individuals' symptoms. These included pulsatilla for women experiencing a "sour taste in the mouth after eating"; "discouragement and sadness"; or "alternating laughing and crying."[14] Describing a case of a nineteen-year-old woman with dysmenorrhea, homeopath E. D. Paine reported the patient cured after remedies of sepia (one dose every eighth day) and pulsatilla (one spoonful every two hours at the recurrence of the periods).[15]

Conventional treatment of uterine hemorrhage during miscarriage or childbirth at this time consisted primarily of external and internal applications of cold water and ice. Homeopaths, believing hemorrhage was a symptom of an "internal malady affecting the whole organism," argued against such treatment. Although ice usually stopped the flow of blood, they believed it would "force" congestion into other organs such as the liver, spleen, and lungs. Patient cases of homeopaths reveal "immediate cessation" of uterine hemorrhage with homeopathic remedies alone. For example, according to the homeopath called to one postparturition woman, the bed and floor was "literally deluged with blood," although she was "buried in ice." After administering "one grain of secale corntum [ergot]," the patient's uterus contracted "at once" and the hemorrhage ceased.[16]

But even in this early period, homeopaths employed mechanical means to "cure" women's so-called diseases. Walter Williamson, author of a section on diseases of "females and children" in Constantine Hering's *Domestic Physician* (1848), claimed he "very frequently" employed the "pessary" in cases when a "well-regulated regime and remedies alone" did not effect a cure.[17] Although more research is needed on homeopathic therapeutics prior to 1860, by that time, there were striking similarities in homeopathic and orthodox ideas and practices in the treatment of women.

Regular physicians employed various therapeutics in the treatment of menstrual irregularities and uterine displacements including: dilating the cervix with sponges, tents, and sounds; the use of electricity or galvanic current in cases assumed to be caused by neuralgia; monthly doses of opiates, sometimes administered hypodermically for pain relief; the placement into the cervix of stem pessaries to support displaced uteri; the application of leeches to the cervix for the treatment of inflammatory congestion of the cervix; bilateral oophorectomy; sitz baths and enemas as "hot as can be borne"; and, failing all else, hysterectomy.[18] In cases where stenosis and particular uterine flexions or displacements were considered the underlying cause of dysmenorrhea, physicians divided the cervix in two places, often inserting a stem pessary to prevent reunion of the cut surfaces. Developed in the 1840s, this procedure was commonly performed until members of the regular profession decried its overuse, and it was largely abandoned by 1880.

Henry Guernsey exemplified the type of practitioner for whom homeopathy was an unqualified alternative to orthodox practice, insisting remedies alone were sufficient in any and all circumstances. But if there ever was a golden age of homeopathy in the United States, where "pure" homeopathy as practiced by Guernsey prevailed, it was relatively short-lived, for his was a minority view as early as the 1860s. Leading homeopaths argued against his notion that homeopathic remedies alone could solve many of women's afflictions.

At a meeting of the Obstetrics Bureau of the AIH in 1869, Guernsey defended himself against critics who challenged his condemnation of appliances such as pessaries and sounds. Guernsey, chair of the Department of Obstetrics at Philadelphia's Hahnemann Medical College and one-time dean of the faculty, enjoyed a national reputation as an educator. Several homeopathic medical schools including Hahnemann Medical College in Philadelphia, Boston University, and New York Medical College and Hospital for Women used Guernsey's obstetrical text in the 1860s and 1870s. Guernsey disdained the use of mechanical appliances in all but a small number of circumstances, arguing that the majority of uterine displacements, including prolapsus, responded to homeopathic medication. Equating pessaries and sounds with the equally harmful and useless therapeutics of heroic medicine, he considered them "barbarous appliances," "useless and degrading as they are disgusting to the female sex," believing they would fall into disuse along with previously denigrated and harmful therapeutics of regular physicians such as cups and blisters, leeches, the lancet, and the cautery.[19]

An angry J. H. Woodbury, a prominent Boston homeopath, said he had recently been at the deathbed of a patient under the care of one of Dr. Guernsey's pupils. After delivery, when the woman's uterus hemorrhaged, the young man "conscientiously stood by" relying on remedies rather than using mechanical pressure to arrest the flow of blood.[20] Woodbury fumed that the student forsook the teachings of common sense in favor of orthodox homeopathic therapeutics. Another physician asked Guernsey if he intended to teach reliance upon internal medication in cases of postpartum hemorrhage when a physician had barely sixty seconds in which to act. Guernsey replied that he had many such cases, and could always arrest the flow with remedies alone. Doctors Baer and Payne discreetly suggested younger members of the profession, lacking an experienced physician's command of the homeopathic materia medica, would have difficulties in this application of homeopathic law. Another individual agreed—in the saving of a life, he said, a physician is justified in the use of any expedient, "regular, irregular, and defective." There is perhaps not one man in five hundred that has the ability to select the proper remedy that Dr. Guernsey has . . . I am compelled to resort to other expedients than medicines. If he needs them not, so much the better." But one less politic physician argued that Guernsey promoted bad medical practice, saying he would not like to have young men sent out from school with such notions.[21]

Did Guernsey's colleagues truly believe his claims of success? No one at the meeting disputed them. But his statements seemed utterly fantastic in light of their own experiences attending women dangerously close to death from postpartum hemorrhage.[22] Most likely, Guernsey's colleagues considered him an extremist, whether or not he possessed extraordinary medical skill. By this time, the majority of homeopathic physicians considered his teachings inappropriate and even dangerous. However, while most homeopaths agreed with Guernsey's critics regarding proper procedure in life-threatening situations, they disagreed on the appropriateness of a host of other procedures such as specular or digital vaginal exams, localized application of medicines, cauterization of the womb in cases of ulceration of the cervix, and the use of mechanical supports such as pessaries.

Although the *Organon* did not mention specific procedures or therapeutic tools such as pessaries, it supported the use of mechanical intervention or topical application of medicines in particular circumstances.[23] Yet much was left to the interpretation of individual physicians, and some homeopaths viewed these methods as examples of an aggressive and interfering style associated with the allopathic school. The overuse of pessaries and other mechanical and topical medications to treat uterine malpositions, menstrual irregularities, and underdevelopment of the uterus was cited by homeopaths (and conservative regulars) as examples of therapeutic excess, creating more problems than they solved. Although homeopaths faulted regular physicians for such improper uterine therapeutics and accused them of contributing to rather than meliorating the sufferings of women, homeopathic physicians often employed the very same tools and procedures.[24]

Ruben Ludlam reported an 1860 case of dysmenorrhea in a twenty-one-year-old married woman, suffering from what she described as "intense neuralgic pains located in the uterine, lumbar, and ishiatic regions."[25] After "six weeks of faithful treatment," using only homeopathic remedies, Ludlam requested and received permission from the patient to perform a vaginal examination. Upon examination, he found a constricted area close to the uterus, and over the course of the next several weeks, Ludlam employed uterine sounds, pessaries, and dilators or sponge-tents to relieve the stricture. Remarking on the chronic nature of the case and the suffering involved, Ludlam noted that the woman had been treated by five or six "eminent" physicians," both homeopathic and regular, in different parts of the country without success. One reason for their failure, he suggested, was lack of a correct diagnosis. Only one physician had proposed a vaginal examination, and the patient refused. In this case, as well as the one reported by Thomas Comstock, patients had expectations of homeopathic care that were different from their regular doctors. Comstock's patient informed him that although the remedies prescribed by her former physician had done her no good, she was satisfied with his rigorousness in selecting them, as he had "studied the materia medica from one to three hours to find the true remedy."[26] She believed her former physician had behaved in an appropriate manner, conforming to her own understanding of proper homeopathic practice; and despite the failure of his treatment, she was reluctant to let go of a firm belief in the correctness of his actions. And in Ludlam's opinion, his patient's confidence in using homeopathic remedies alone to effect a change in her condition exceeded his own. He seemed slightly defensive about turning to mechanical measures, and was careful to report that he did not resort to such means until approximately twenty-four hours in advance of her third menstrual period while under his care.

Having previously been treated by homeopaths who did not require vaginal examinations, Comstock's and Ludlam's patients were surprised at their insistence on the procedure. As homeopathic therapeutics grew more similar to conventional treatment and practitioners competed for patients, some homeopaths sought ways to differentiate themselves from regular doctors. Patients' assumptions and expectations often influenced their choice of procedures.

A homeopath practicing in the textile city of Lynn, Massachusetts, reported a conversation with a young woman troubled by leukorrhea. She said she knew hundreds of women and girls, sewing machine operators in the mills, who were bothered by the same condition.[27] She was pleasantly surprised that she did not have to submit to a local examination, and spread the word among her coworkers. The physician stated that many of the mill workers came to him for treatment when they learned they could be treated without undergoing vaginal examinations.[28] Homeopath James Tyler Kent said that he made no vaginal examination in the case of of Miss A.W., a patient he diagnosed as having an ovarian tumor so large it resembled a nine-month pregnancy. The patient, an Irish housemaid, told Dr. Kent she came to him because she heard a local examination would not be made.[29] Another homeopath took on a patient who had been treated for painful menstruation by an allopathic doctor whose "trade methods" (douches), he said, resulted in leukorrhea. The homeopathic physician said he refused to make a vaginal examination in part because "I desired . . . to appear as to my method, different in every respect to her allopathic adviser."[30]

Local examination and especially use of the speculum were criticized by some homeopaths and regulars who believed the procedure brought previously hidden parts of the anatomy into view, encouraging topical applications of medications as well as mechanical and surgical interference. Hahnemannians and older traditional homeopaths believed such examinations were unnecessary aids for the physician in choosing a homeopathic remedy. Those who resisted the "speculum craze" argued that having convinced a woman that the procedure was necessary, the onus was on the physician to "find" pathology even where none existed, thus justifying the procedure.[31] But lack of consensus in addition to discussions on the use of specula, vaginal examinations, and localized treatment characterized physicians' practices. And like their male colleagues, women homeopaths were divided on questions of what constituted proper homeopathic practice, with the majority sharing men's enthusiasm for mechanical and topical adjuvants.

Anna Manning Comfort specialized in women's diseases, practicing first in Norwich, Connecticut, then New York City, and later in Syracuse, New York. Almost all the seventy-four patients she treated in 1867 received medications applied to the vagina, cervix, and uterus. In the majority of cases, Comfort used topical applications of red powder dressing (possibly cinchona), and less frequently, caustic silver, nitric acid, and idoform. Fourteen of Dr. Comfort's patients underwent leeching and/or the vaginal insertion of sounds, tents, and bongies (sponges) impregnated with slippery elm bark.[32]

Eliza Cook, an 1880 graduate of New York Medical College and Hospital for Women, was consulted by a woman who had been married eleven years, yet was unable to become pregnant. Upon examination Dr. Cook found Mrs. G.'s uterus to be "not quite two inches long, with thin walls, a tortuous cavity, and the body shriveled and rigid." Her management of the case consisted of dilating the "twisted" canal for three days in a row after which she inserted a short, rubber-stem pessary. Her patient was to wear it for one month, but "whether from constipation or some thoughtless movement," it was "thrown out." Dr. Cook inserted a larger stem. For one year, the pessary was worn and replaced at regular intervals. At the end of this time Dr. Cook believed that Mrs. G's womb "had grown straight and to a normal size," so she could wear a pessary with a longer stem than her present device. After an additional six months, "to fortify against a relapse," the pessary was removed. Dr. Cook said she did not hear from her patient again until she called to consult the doctor on the management of her "confinement" after delivering a healthy boy.[33]

In Boston, members of the Massachusetts Homoeopathic Medical Society discussed their preferences in treating a case of ulceration of the uterus at an 1874 meeting. Dr. Hall, blaming the harsh treatment of the "old school" for a great many cases of uterine diseases, said he used no local applications of any kind. Dr. Bell, a visiting physician from Augusta, Maine, said he seldom used the speculum to confirm or refute a diagnosis, and employed only internal remedies in treatment. Dr. Mercy B. Jackson, one of the first women homeopaths in Boston and a faculty member of the medical school at Boston University, stated that her use of the speculum did not exceed one-third of her uterine cases, and she rejected use of the sound, considering it very dangerous. She noted that she "has never" used caustics or topical applications other than mild castile soap. However, Dr. Krebs stated that he "is in constant use of the speculum" and acknowledged the usefulness of the sound, while Israel Talbot, one of Boston's most prominent homeopaths, considered the occasional use of the speculum very valuable.[34] Homeopaths attending the annual meeting of the AIH in 1876 expressed similarly eclectic views in treating displacements of the uterus. Some advocated hygienic measures or remedies alone, others relied on electricity, local means of scarification, cauterization, astringent lotions, injections, and suppositories. Some physicians chose mechanical means such as pessaries, perineal pads, and abdominal supporters.[35] Most homeopaths doubted that homeopathic remedies alone could effect a cure. By the last third of the century, homeopaths' education, practical experience, and competition for patients broadened the meaning of homeopathy, severely minimizing its distinctiveness as an unequivocal medical alternative. Their eclectic practices caused institutional as well as personal conflict.

Maintaining Homeopathic Identity

Struggling to maintain homeopathy as a unique system, Hahnemannians criticized the work of the majority of their colleagues. But they also realized that to ignore new diagnostic techniques, procedures, and treatment marginalized not only homeopathy, but also their own status as physicians. They understood that the ability to "name" a disease and identify its cause was a powerful new source of authority for physicians. Though some discounted the importance of pathological anatomy and the rise of microscopic pathology in terms of aiding homeopaths in their choice of remedies, most acknowledged their value to the perception of homeopathy as a progressive medical science.[36]

Hahnemannian Sarah J. Millsop, an 1886 graduate of Hahnemann Medical College in Chicago, agreed that even if the homeopathic method of prescribing according to the law of similars did not depend on pathological conditions, ignoring such conditions would come at the expense of ". . . our reputation as a school."[37] Millsop practiced medicine in Bowling Green, Kentucky, and frequently consulted regular physicians whose claims of superior diagnostic abilities she sought to refute. Dr. Millsop stated that among regular physicians as well as the "laity" there was an assumption that homeopaths, while they cured people, knew less than allopaths about the human system or the cause of disease. This impression, she believed, stemmed from the attitudes of some homeopaths who said openly that to name the disease was of no consequence. Their zeal in basing treatment on observed symptoms, according to Millsop, overshadowed the importance to the patient of knowing the name and nature of the disorder. Millsop said she was dedicated to homeopathic remedies prescribed on the basis of symptoms, but argued that the ability to diagnose and name disease would increase the confidence of patients, enhance the physician's own satisfaction by understanding a case in its entirety, and elevate the reputation of homeopaths as a group. Her increased diagnostic abilities, she said, allowed her to meet any "old school" doctor in consultation without fear.[38]

Homeopath Mary Brinkman felt her task of healing was complicated by the "fine line" she had to walk as a homeopathic physician. She expressed frustration at the difficulty of maintaining her identity as an "avowed" homeopathic physician, striving to keep pace with the advance of medical science without "violating the 'tenets' of homoeopathy in daily practice." Brinkman acknowledged that physicians were deluged by discoveries of microbes and bacilli in the causation of disease, proposals to inoculate against infectious diseases such as smallpox, yellow fever, and cholera, and by an increase in the latest surgical procedures. She was convinced that the notion and dogma of localized disease and treatment was faulty, and that the homeopathic gynecologist should delve deeper into the realm of preventive medicine, rather than be sidetracked by the varieties of new discoveries and theories. But the ascendancy of surgery as a specialty, rather than attention to prevention, was the primary factor in causing gynecologists to turn away from the ineffective therapeutics of pessaries and caustics.[39]

Gynecological Surgery and Homeopathy

As early as 1850, surgeons had developed techniques to repair successfully vesico-vaginal and rectal fistulas, and to remove "diseased ovaries" (ovariotomy or oophorectomy). By 1880, dramatic advances in surgery including widespread use of anesthesia and antisepsis reduced the pain of surgery and perils of infection. An ample supply of patients with similar diseases, more willing to be hospitalized, allowed doctors to perform surgeries under controlled conditions. By 1890, Caesarean sections and hysterectomies were not uncommon. And although this turn of events eliminated the worst abuses of mechanical interventionist therapeutics, it created new problems.[40]

Homeopaths were slower than regular physicians to embrace surgical therapeutics. According to William Tod Helmuth, one of the brightest lights in homeopathic surgery late in the century, early homeopaths referred surgical patients to regular physicians. When the AMA forbade consultation with homeopaths, the specialty of surgery within homeopathy began to develop. Chair of surgery and later dean of New York Homoeopathic Medical College, Helmuth perfected his techniques in Europe and pioneered the surgical art among homeopathic physicians. He blamed surgery's retarded pace on the "great professors" of homeopathy who, in their excessive zeal for Hahnemann's law, exhibited a "careless disregard" of surgery, stressing internal remedies instead. "In earlier times," said Helmuth, "there was an opprobrium, 'No surgery; no surgeons among the homoeopathists.'" Even today [1893], he said, homeopaths undervalue surgery as a means of propagating the interests of and securing a place of honor for the profession. While Hahnemann did not discount the value of surgery in particular circumstances, his emphasis on internal medication coupled with the low status and risks of surgery caused homeopaths to avoid it. By the late nineteenth century, however, Helmuth and other young, progressive homeopaths considered homeopathic remedies important complementary therapy for surgical patients, hastening healing, and palliating pain.[41]

While older homeopaths may indeed have been slow to realize the value of surgery in the enhancement of professional prestige and influence, others debated the appropriateness of particular surgical procedures in individual cases. However, by the last decade of the century, if not before, most agreed on surgery's legitimacy in homeopathic therapeutics and its role in enhancing the prestige of the profession. In a lecture to students on homeopathic philosophy, James T. Kent complained: "You know how we are maligned and lied about. You have heard it said about some strict homoeopath, 'He tried to set a broken leg with the c.m.[centesimal] potency of Mercury. What a poor fool!'" Kent, the acknowledged leader of the strictest Hahnemannians at the turn of the century, cautioned his students "always" to discriminate between the internal and external causes of disease: "It is folly to give medicine for a lacerated wound, to attempt to close up a deep wound with a dose of remedy."[42] Sarah J. Millsop, an 1886 graduate of Hahnemann Medical College of Chicago and vice president of the AIH in 1899, expressed pride that her profession numbered many skilled and prestigious surgeons. As the only female physician within hundreds of miles of her home in Bowling Green, Kentucky, Millsop enjoyed a large practice in gynecology. But with few homeopathic physicians in her part of the state, as Dr. Millsop put it, she worked in the midst of a "den" of allopaths. Although not a surgeon herself, Millsop believed the skillful accomplishments and fine reputations of homeopathic surgeons increased her credibility and standing among those regular doctors as well as her patients.[43]

Despite the earlier generation's reluctance to embrace surgical solutions, individual homeopathic surgeons adopted antiseptic and aseptic procedures around the same time as regulars, and were acknowledged for notable surgical achievements. In 1876, William Todd Helmuth performed one of the first antiseptic operations (ovariotomy) in the United States.[44] San Francisco homeopath, James Ward, was a recognized authority on abdominal surgery; and his wife, Florence Nightingale Ward, was lauded in 1894 and 1895 for six-teen successful vaginal hysterectomies and twelve cases involving the removal of uterine fibroid tumors.[45] The primary difference between homeopathic and regular surgeons was the use of homeopathic remedies both before and after surgeries to reduce shock and promote healing.

Hospital reports provide added dimension to the state of gynecological surgery in the last decades of the century. In 1886 William Todd Helmuth founded a private hospital accommodating about twenty patients on East Twelfth Street in New York City. The 1887 biannual report of Helmuth House listed sixty-one operations. Three-quarters of the surgical procedures were performed on women, including mastectomy, hysterectomy, ovariotomy, repair of fistulas, perineorrhaphy (repair of perineum), and trachelorrhaphy (repair of the cervix). Out of nine deaths, five were women who had under-gone hysterectomy and/or ovariotomy. The report stressed that high mortality excluded hysterectomy from the list of justifiable operations, except in extreme cases, noting Dr. Helmuth's mortality rates were average for ovari-otomy—about 20 percent.[46]

Unfortunately, the broad categories and vague language of hospital reports are short on specifics. Most did not differentiate between patients' age, sex, and race or list specific surgical procedures. Surgeons at Massachusetts Homoeopathic Hospital performed 1,185 surgeries in 1898—almost half for what were termed "diseases of the genito-urinary system." Yet we know noth-ing of the patients or their specific surgeries. Fortunately, surviving case records for these years offered more details.[47] An analysis of 111 cases involv-ing adults admitted to the surgical ward of Massachusetts Homoeopathic Hos-pital during July and November 1897, involved eighty-nine women and twenty-two men. Records show that while two men underwent castration, a majority were treated for appendicitis, cysts, abscesses, and tumors unrelated to sexual organs. Some job-related injuries required surgery, and one involved removing a bullet from the shoulder of a Boston sea captain. Among the women, 60 percent underwent surgeries for gynecological problems, including repair of lacerated cervix and/or perineum (18); hysterectomy (13); curetting of uterus (13); mastectomy (6); ovariotomy (3); and myomectomy or removal of fibroid tumors (2).[48]

Although the development of new and successful surgical procedures pro-vided physicians and patients with possible solutions to previously untreatable conditions, some homeopaths and regulars alike viewed the surgical trend with suspicion.[49] During the 1895 meeting of the AIH, one physician noticed several colleagues deserting a gynecology meeting in favor of another on obstetrics. When asked why they had left, one physician responded: "The Gynaecological Bureau is simply a surgical bureau. There's nothing going on of especial interest to general practitioners." Another added: "It would seem as if there is nothing to be done for the relief of suffering women but some sort of an operation."[50] The attitudes of these doctors were common among regu-lars as well, and reflected professional rivalry in addition to uncertainty over newly developing models of professional identity and medical specialization.[51]

Physicians in general struggled to elevate their profession, in their own eyes as well as the public's. Seeking to stabilize the boundaries of their special-ties, they engaged in a considerable amount of faultfinding. According to gynecologists, lack of skill in the use of forceps by generalists and obstetricians resulted in many perineal and cervical lacerations. Physician accoucheurs often realized their role in obstetrical problems, but the demands and duties of general practice often prevented them from acting in the best interests of their maternity patients. They often neglected postpartum examinations, and failed to diagnose and properly repair lacerations.

With the superiority typical of gynecologists of that era, Sarah J. Millsop claimed that there would be less "of a certain kind of work for gynecologists to do" if obstetricians did their work better.[52] A gynecological surgeon at Buffalo Homoeopathic Hospital agreed with her. He had observed large numbers of women with lacerations of the perineum or cervix dating from parturition. Blaming such problems on "older" practitioners who failed to recognize them and on the "average obstetrician of smaller communities," he said those physi-cians remained unaware of the large percentage of their parturient patients who eventually came to the operating table.[53] Sarah J. Lee, a homeopathic gynecologist in Rochester, New York, in 1889, estimated that lacerations existed in 20 to 30 percent in primiparas and from 5 to 10 percent in multi-paras. "Still," she said, "there are men who claim to have enjoyed a large obstetrical practice for years, without ever having had a perineum lacerate."[54] Dr. Lee's reference to "men" may have indicated she considered male physi-cians more neglectful than female doctors in diagnosing perineal or vaginal lacerations. But men did comprise the majority of the profession, and in fact women physicians were subject to the same criticism.

In the presence of doubting colleagues at the 1880 meeting of the AIH, "Mrs. Dr. Cook of Chicago" claimed to have delivered two thousand women without one case of a lacerated perineum.[55] One physician questioned whether her patients could have had problems unknown to her, but Dr. Cook denied that possibility, and spoke of her attention to prevention. Long before her patients entered labor, Dr. Cook examined them, prescribing hygienic measures; and, although she was slightly embarrassed to say it, applied non-homeopathic doses of belladonna cerate to the cervix prior to labor. In addition, she insisted her careful and thorough follow-up care revealed any problems missed during deliveries. Dr. Cook's response reflected a notable difference between male and female physicians in general—women's more active involvement and interest in preventive medicine. Like women regulars, homeopaths frequently stressed the hygiene, fitness, proper dress, and prescriptions of prevention.

During a discussion of obstetrics at the annual meeting of the AIH in 1894, Dr. Jane Culver said she appreciated the valuable suggestions relating to "abnormalities of maternity" placed before the group by her male colleagues, but urged consideration of another side—the regulation of diet, dress, and exercise, both physical and mental.[56] Sarah J. Millsop argued for a broader definition of prevention, including earlier attention to the parturient woman's behavior, examination of women's nonreproductive organs, and the importance of psychology to a patient's sense of well-being.[57] Millsop criticized physicians' negligent therapeutics in treating mammary abscesses occurring during lactation. Doctors ignored problems with breasts, she said, because they did not come under the rubric of "reproductive organs," which were of greater interest to medical men. Millsop deplored the practice of lancing mammary abscesses after "ignorant untaught nurses" applied various "greasy, dirty-looking applications" in a vain attempt to prevent them from forming. And Hannah Tyler Wilcox of Chicago encouraged her colleagues to investigate the physiological and psychological benefits of oxytocic electricity to obviate the need for drugs and forceps during delivery and prevent postpartum hemorrhage. "It gives courage to the patient in feeling that something is being done to relieve her suffering."[58] But while gender played a role in discussions of prevention, changes in the location of medical treatment intensified the professional gulf between general practitioners, obstetricians, and gynecologists, subsuming differences between homeopaths and regulars.

Shifting Locations of Medical Care

During the last third of the nineteenth century, the rapidly growing urban middle class looked more favorably upon hospitalization as an appropriate and safe venue for medical care. The unique opportunities of urban physicians for hospital work contrasted with most rank and file practitioners, even specialists. Speaking at a meeting of the AIH in 1903, homeopath gynecologist Florence Ward contrasted "private work" with "hospital work" in the rates of infection following repair of ruptured perineums and lesions occurring during childbirth. Ward claimed that the maternal mortality in private practice doubled from that of half a century ago, with infection the rule rather than the exception. Dr. Ward favored hospitalization of parturient mothers, believing competent accoucheurs would reduce the number of perineal and cervical lacerations and that skilled surgeons could handle necessary surgical repairs.[59]

Several individuals agreed with her, finding "poor surgery and poorer obstetrics" undertaken in a patient's home by an obstetrician or general practitioner largely responsible for the abysmal picture of maternal mortality. Reflecting on the growing technological complexity of childbirth, homeopath Margaret Koch declared it impossible for any obstetrician to oversee the administration of anesthesia while simultaneously doing good surgical work. One homeopath, defending competent "private work," said he employed trained nurses to aid him in the repair of lacerations and follow-up care. In fact, he would not attend a case, he said, where a patient did not agree to have one. This provoked a sardonic response from someone who pointed to the folly of such expectations in rural practice. After an eleven-mile horseback ride on muddy country roads, far from any skilled assistance, he could not enter a one-room cabin with a woman laboring and announce, "You have got to have a trained nurse or I will not touch the case."[60] Clearly, most physicians practiced medicine in a context very different from that of elite, urban doctors, whose work in hospitals or homes of the middle and upper classes allowed more control of circumstances.

By the 1890s, many obstetricians became proficient in surgical repair of lacerations, and in curette and dilation of the uterus following a miscarriage or abortion. Charges of meddlesome midwifery had led to significant reforms. Physicians attending the annual AIH meeting in 1894 considered premature breaking of the waters, hurrying to assist nature with forceps or drugs, and failure to repair immediately a lacerated perineum poor obstetrical practice. By the end of the century, concerns focused on gynecological surgery, eclipsing attention to the perceived and/or real inadequacies of obstetricians and general practitioners.

The public and many leading physicians reproached gynecologists for excessive zeal in extirpating women's sexual organs. Although logically homeopaths should have been the most conservative surgeons, that was not the case, as evidenced by criticisms from their homeopathic colleagues. Hahnemannian gynecologist Lizzie Gray Gutherz cautioned fellow homeopaths to forsake the "brilliant feats of knife and chisel" for the "more enduring though less alluring" achievements of homeopathic medication. Reminding them of their special mission on behalf of women, she said that when Hahnemann evolved the law of similia, he gave to "tired, tried, misused, oftentimes mismanaged woman a host of steadfast friends whose name is legion."[61] Early on, older, traditional homeopaths such as Henry Guernsey cautioned homeopaths to demand more of themselves than simply resorting to surgical operations. Younger, late-nineteenth-century Hahnemannians and many women homeopaths were allies in calling for more self-control by homeopathic surgeons.

In 1896, *The Medical Century*, a respected and widely read homeopathic periodical, published a plea for a return to remedies in gynecology, criticizing the current medical literature for devoting the most space to local surgical and instrumental treatments, while including only a few references to homeopathic remedies. The writer believed that a good family physician should turn cases over to good gynecological or abdominal surgeons only when remedies failed to rectify problems.[62] As he saw it, homeopathy was most effective as a first line of defense in the hands of general practitioners.

As Martin Pernick has artfully shown, the nineteenth-century's "calculus of safety"—a careful measuring of benefits and risks to patients—originated largely as a response to criticism of heroic therapy by advocates of natural healing. Although it emerged within debates over the use of anesthesia to control pain during surgery, it broadened the thinking of physicians in determining whether the "disease" or the "cure" was the lesser evil.[63] Homeopathy played a principal role in the development of this "calculus"; yet, homeopathic physicians had not been immune to the spirit of medical progress, the rise of specialties, and increased authority generated by the spectacular rise in the prestige of surgery. By the end of the century, ovariotomies and/or hysterectomies had become standard procedures for treating ovarian and uterine cysts and tumors, pelvic inflammation caused by abscesses, cancer, and infection of the fallopian tubes, ovaries, or uterus. Within this context, and in response to rising criticism, homeopaths as well as regulars reexamined their ideas on the circumstances justifying an ovariotomy or hysterectomy.

Conservative Surgery and Preventive Medicine

Women physicians—regulars as well as homeopaths—became outspoken critics of excesses in gynecological surgery. At a meeting of the AIH in 1894, Hannah Tyler Wilcox expressed her hope that as more women became doctors, they would teach conservatism in the treatment of their sex. Wilcox framed her plea for such a turn of events on the inequity of the present situation, and on the discrimination she perceived in the treatment of the sexes. Unlike women, Wilcox said, men do not get unsexed. "Do they [men] not suffer disease of the testicles and sexual organs from gonorrhea and syphilis? Is it not that sex who are mainly responsible for these evils which afflict women? Do we make eunuchs of men?" She argued that not every headache or backache of which men complained resulted in the ablation and extirpation of their sexual apparatus. Some individuals took considerable offense at some of Dr. Wilcox's statements. Defending himself against the charge of too-frequent sexual surgery, Dr. Lee claimed that, as a specialist with patients from all over the country, he naturally performed a considerable number of surgeries. Lee adamantly replied that while "I operate often, . . . I do not unsex every woman who comes to me."[64]

Some feminist historians have viewed professional disputes over radical surgical procedures and the "unsexing" of women as examples of male misogyny, casting women in the role of victim.[65] However, it was not unusual for patients to request removal of ovaries when aware that such surgery provided a permanent means of preventing conception. A Philadelphia homeopath attending a woman during her first parturition resorted to a craniotomy to extract the child. At the woman's second pregnancy, he performed a Caesarean section, and "at the urgent request of the patient and of her husband, I consented to remove the ovaries at the operation in order to prevent the recurrence of pregnancy."[66] Some physicians believed women were only too willing to have their ovaries removed, that the dread of having children had done much to make the procedure popular. Although the terms "oophorectomy" and "ovariotomy" were often used interchangeably, surgeons gradually began to distinguish beween them. "Oophorectomy" as promoted by Georgia surgeon Robert Battey referred to the removal of healthy-appearing ovaries due to acute menstrual problems or various types of nervous conditions. "Ovariotomy" was most often associated with Lawson Tait's technique—the removal of Fallopian tubes and ovaries that appeared to be diseased. One physician claimed that the "fair sex" was quite carried away with the idea of oophorectomy, and upon the slightest provocation would not only submit to the operation themselves, but also would try to induce their friends to do likewise.[67] Although this physician implied women's interest in oophorectomy was a fad, reproduction and childbearing were fraught with difficulty. Many women described lifelong "womb troubles," dating their gynecological problems from improperly managed or difficult childbirths. The use of pessaries and forceps, caustic topical applications to the genitalia, and the invasiveness of instruments to reposition "displaced" uteri, all methods designed to cure problems, added to them. For many women, surgery seemed the least harmful and most successful solution to long-standing debility and/or the prevention of pregnancy.[68]

Sensitive to criticism of excesses in gynecological surgery and eager to learn about his patients' quality of life, one homeopath in 1903 sent a questionnaire to 163 female surgical patients. Eighty-six had undergone hysterectomies, eighteen ovariotomies, and the rest had myomectomies or curetting of the uterus. Dr. Emerson wanted to know if his patients had been "restored to life of ordinary usefulness and activity proper to their age and circumstances, or are they merely physical wrecks of another type?" Of the 124 responses to the question on whether the women would undergo the operation again, four were in doubt, five said "no," and 115 said "yes."[69]

By the last decade of the nineteenth century, many doctors—male and female, homeopathic and regular—argued for reform in gynecological surgery. In large part, the debate was between two generations of physicians. Older, Paris-trained doctors insisted therapeutic decisions should be grounded in physiological knowledge and bedside observation of patients; while younger physicians gave greater credence to laboratory knowledge. The latter viewed surgery as more scientific than general medicine, with its diagnoses and surgical decisions based on the latest discoveries in anatomy, physiology, chemistry, and pathology. In part, the debate was driven by beliefs in the racial superiority of western European cultures and in women's proper role in society. Social and cultural conservatives denounced procedures that would preclude Anglo American women from fulfilling their maternal duty to propagate the "superior" race.[70]

However, reform in gynecology was also driven by yet another professional turf battle. As Nancy Theriot argues, gynecologists, alienists (psychiatrists), and neurologists debated competing theories of the origin of disease.[71] Their assumptions regarding the nature of women's mental disease and "nervousness" demonstrate how professional, public, and personal interests influence concepts of disease.

Competing Theories of Disease

At the 1894 AIH meeting, Dr. Pratt reprimanded Hannah Wilcox for her ignorance of the frequency of castration on male patients—not only for men with "legitimate troubles," he said, but also for "mental conditions."[72] Pratt's statement demonstrates that some physicians viewed sexual surgery in the treatment of mental disorders as an "illegitimate" use of the surgical art. Their opinion had less to do with concerns about women being unfairly targeted for such surgery, than it did with specialists' changing ideas on the origin of disease.

Hannah Wilcox noted with annoyance that doctors rarely used "reflex conditions" to explain illness in men. Popular in the mid- and late-nineteenth century, the "reflex irritation" model of disease assumed an intimate link between a woman's sexual organs, especially the uterus, and every other part of her body. Theoretically, a "diseased womb" wreaked its havoc via the "sympathetic nerve," the pathway for pathological responses in other organs or mental faculties.[73] But late in the nineteenth century, competing theories on the origin of mental and nervous disease gained acceptance among a number of prominent homeopaths and regulars, commensurate with their growing interest in neurology and psychiatry.

Alienists and neurologists believed psychological and environmental, or situational factors, in addition to the physiological, caused nervousness or mental illness. They believed disorders of the nervous system, not "diseased" sexual organs, produced insanity, neurasthenia, hysteria, and epilepsy. Their common ground with gynecologists lay in the assumption of gender differences regarding illness. The specialties assumed and explained women's essential difference from men not only (or even primarily) due to their interest in building specialized practices in gynecology, neurology, or psychiatry but also because of general sociocultural views of gender distinction.[74] Physicians, however, assuming "male" to be the standard measure, evolved explanations for women's differences based on deviations from this standard, according to the internal logic and accumulated knowledge within their medical fields.[75]

Many gynecologists only reluctantly abandoned theories privileging their areas of expertise, training, and education. Homeopathic gynecologist James Ward stated that "in order to stamp out insanity, I am strongly induced to believe in the legal castration of the individual of either sex, who is the unfortunate victim of this hereditary curse."[76] Yet despite Ward's "egalitarian" views, women were rendered sterile more often. Women physicians, including many gynecologists, contributed to the discourse on competing views of causation almost entirely in opposition to the gynecological perspective.[77] They took exception to the idea that a disturbance in the genital organs caused every backache, headache, or depression in women, promoting an etiology based on women's role in society. They argued that women's domestic environment, narrow life choices, the "monotony of work and thought" in the roles of wife and mother, and the unremitting labor of working-class women, were the primary causes of mental breakdowns.[78]

For example, Boston homeopath Harriet Clisby believed many cases of serious nervous diseases and other maladies among women of all classes originated from lack of education, as well as vital and interesting work.[79] According to Mary Brinkman, women's nervous diseases derived from violations of proper hygiene, dress, diet, and moral behavior. As a specialist in women's diseases, she urged her colleagues to investigate a range of therapeutic possibilities, including hygiene, mechanics, chemistry, physiological research, microscopic investigation, surgery, and application of the properly selected homeopathic remedy. Addressing the Alumnae Association of New York Medical College and Hospital for Women in New York City in 1889, Brinkman envisioned a narrower scope for gynecology, questioning not only the "so-called" local diseases of the pelvic organs but also the entire dogma of local disease. She complained that the terms "neurasthenia" and "nervous exhaustion . . . fall glibly from the lips of our young women," asking "What is the gynaecologist to do? Shall he resort to the latest medical 'fad,' and remove the ovaries? Cut off elongated ligaments, stitch the retroverted uterus to the abdominal wall, etc.?" Calling these "bungling," last-resort measures both ineffectual and dangerous, Dr. Brinkman argued that, "Mutilation is not cure."[80] While not rejecting the idea of reflex disturbances, she believed them to be centrifugal as well as centripetal, and encouraged particular attention to the emotional sphere, especially in the selection of remedies.[81]

The greater interest in and broader definition of preventive medicine of alienists and neurologists led to dissatisfaction with the narrow construction of gynecology, causing gynecologists to neglect social and environmental influences that could identify and extirpate "diseased" sexual organs. Women homeopaths and regular physicians resisted explanations that limited educational, intellectual, and career choices (especially their own) based upon physiology. Few entered the predominately male professional terrain of gynecological surgery, perhaps finding it less appealing philosophically as well as less accessible.[82]

For physicians like Florence Ward whose interests and ambition led them to become surgeons, the adoption of conservative, organ-saving methods enabled them to pursue their professional goals although they found "local lesion" an unsatisfactory and incomplete explanation for the cause of disease. Ward, a leading West Coast homeopath and proponent of conservatism in sexual surgery, studied gynecology with leading surgeons in Germany, Austria, and France. She was familiar with the observations of physicians in Paris and research in Vienna, Berlin, and Luzerne showing the ovary to be a secretory organ whose importance to overall health was equal to its role in reproduction. Whereas her husband advocated aggressive surgery, Florence Ward considered the preservation of organs a higher surgical art. The conservative ethic tempered the earlier masculine vision of the bold, brilliant, and daring surgeon. Florence Ward spoke of the still unknown "mysteries of the vital processes taking place within the ovary," and argued that with "delicate and careful plastic work upon the tubes and ovaries, we can preserve them functionally perfect." Speaking of the "wholesale ablation" of ovaries as a solution to pelvic disease and pain, as well as "countless reflex and nervous disturbances that afflict womankind," Ward said the "wholesale mutilation and production of sterility" had not brought the perfect cure. The most important, perhaps only benefit of over-zealous abdominal surgery lay in increased understanding of the ovary, its functions, and its various pathological lesions.[83]

In 1911 Florence Ward founded a private hospital in San Francisco, where perfection of conservative surgical techniques and careful attention to patients in their pre- and postoperative stages would, she hoped, result in low mortality rates and rapid restoration of patients' health. Reporting on three years' surgical work from 1911 to 1914, Ward was quite pleased with her results. Although sixty-five out of seventy-nine patients with uterine fibroids had undergone hysterectomies, out of twenty-eight patients with ovarian cysts, none had a double oophorectomy. In eighty-two cases of diseased fallopian tubes, more than two-thirds retained one ovary and/or fallopian tube. In no cases did women diagnosed with uterine displacements or prolapses receive hysterectomies or oophorectomies.[84]

As a homeopathic surgeon, Ward used remedies in conjunction with surgical techniques to treat ovarian disease, but cautioned physicians to use them appropriately. The physician should recognize the spheres, surgical or medicinal, and shape treatment accordingly. Inappropriate use of remedies, she said, would not only waste valuable time but also throw homeopathic methods into disrepute.[85] Clearly, Ward was not referring to the majority of her colleagues, whose gynecological therapeutics in the decades leading up to the turn of the century were not essentially different from those of the regular school. In their training and in their different views of gynecological surgery, James and Florence Ward epitomized modern, progressive medical opinion and practice. It seemed only a matter of time before the divisions between homeopathic and regular medicine would disappear.

While women patients often had expectations of homeopathic care that differed significantly from the therapeutics of regulars, they were often disappointed. By the middle of the nineteenth century, many homeopaths had begun to use traditional homeopathic remedies in conjunction with procedures and therapeutic devices associated with regular physicians. Although homeopaths defended these practices, arguing that Hahnemann himself approved of mechanical intervention or topical applications in certain circumstances, it became increasingly difficult for homeopaths to maintain a distinctive identity. Along with the growth of specialties, especially gynecological surgery, homeopaths resembled regular physicians in many ways—a development that was both welcomed and condemned by members of the profession. By the end of the 1800s, the only homeopaths advocating a primary reliance on internal remedies were a small minority of Hahnemannians, believing they alone were the homeopathic torchbearers of the next century.

Chapter 6

The Transformation of American Medicine and the Decline of Homeopathy, 1890–1920

In 1899, REFLECTING THE WILL of the majority of its members, the American Institute of Homeopathy changed its definition of a homeopathic physician to "one who adds to his knowledge of medicine a special knowledge of homeopathic therapeutics. All that pertains to medicine is his, by inheritance, by tradition, by right."[1] An 1898 issue of the *Cresset*, a student publication of the homeopathic New York Medical College and Hospital for Women, defined homeopathy not as a school of medicine but a "reform in one of its departments—the sphere of therapeutics. Homeopathy "has no new anatomy, chemistry, physiology, obstetrics, surgery, pathology, hygiene, or sanitation. It shares all these things with the allopathic school."[2] By the turn of the century, homeopaths had refashioned their profession as a therapeutic field, supplemental and "additional" to general medicine.[3] However, the choice of the profession's leaders to emphasize homeopathy's similarities to mainstream medicine was not a rejection of its separate identity. Rather, it revealed a homeopathic profession endeavoring to keep pace with the new scientific and professional developments of the Progressive movement.

Within the culture of a new professionalism characterizing the Progressive Era in American history, American universities standardized training for careers, producing professional experts whose voices of authority discouraged independent evaluation by untrained individuals and amateur social reformers.[4] As new and existing professions sought to increase their power and prestige, the medical profession set the standard by reforming medical education, aligning with the states to reinstitute licensing regulations, and creating a national political base. A pioneer in public relations strategy, a reorganized and strengthened AMA succeeded in projecting a favorable public image,

successfully resisting threats to physician autonomy by various forms of contract practice advanced by hospitals, benevolent societies, fraternal lodges,
and industries, as well as campaigns for compulsory health insurance organized by labor leaders. These reforms decreased the number of physicians (one
of the AMA's major goals), while increasing physician autonomy, social status, income, and regulations for practice. By the end of the Progressive Era,
American medicine had truly become "organized medicine."[5]

The transformation of American medicine had a decided effect on women's
homeopathic education and professional opportunities. Like their male colleagues, most women considered themselves physicians first and homeopaths
second. By integrating the ideals and practices of scientific medicine into
homeopathy, they blurred their separate identity as homeopathic physicians.
At the same time, however, a minority of women homeopaths became leaders
in organizations to preserve and propagate the traditional or "pure" homeopathy of Samuel Hahnemann. Although few in number, Hahnemannian women
comprised a larger percentage of such organizations compared with women in
the AIH and the profession as a whole, finding professional advantages and
personal meaning in their advocacy of an older, less technological approach to
healing.

Although marginal to mainstream medicine as well as the larger homeopathic profession, Hahnemannians incorporated values traditionally linked
with the feminine, blending them with a kind of homeopathy its advocates
considered "ultra-scientific," intellectually rigorous, and difficult to master.
Considering themselves the elite of the homeopathic profession, Hahnemannians constructed a separate professional arena in which women had equal
access to status, professional opportunities, and leadership roles at a time
when they were forced to the margins of the mainstream medical profession.[6]

Consolidation and Reform

In the 1880s and 1890s, the AMA supported state legislation establishing
qualifications for medical education and practice, as well as the formation of
examining boards for the licensure of physicians. In locations such as New
York and Massachusetts where the political influence of homeopaths was
strong, separate boards of regulars, eclectics, and homeopaths examined candidates from their own schools. Recognizing, however, that integrated boards
were more effective in controlling entrance into the profession, regulars promoted boards composed of physicians from all three groups.[7] Questions considered unfair to graduates of homeopathic schools were typically replaced
with those testing their specific knowledge in homeopathic materia medica

and therapeutics. Homeopaths recognized the benefits of cooperating with regular physicians in establishing composite boards. Similar to regulars, students in homeopathic and eclectic schools were educated in the basic sciences. They believed in the power of drugs (however variously defined) to effect cures, and were eager to distinguish themselves from practitioners of the newly popular but unscientific "drugless cults" of osteopathy, chiropractic, and Christian Science.[8] By 1924, only five states maintained separate boards. Thirty-three states had single, composite boards, requiring graduates to be competent in all areas of medicine.[9]

As reforms in medical education altered the curricula of schools with new subjects and courses, examinations stressed knowledge in the basic medical sciences and clinical subjects. Over time, homeopathic materia medica and therapeutics became a less important part of the curricula of homeopathic schools struggling to conform to the new educational standards. During the last third of the nineteenth century, homeopathy gradually lost currency as a separate school of medicine.[10]

In 1903, believing that science alone—rather than abstract theory—would determine physicians' practices, the AMA changed the code of ethics that had been a key source of antagonism between the professions for much of the nineteenth century. The revised code gave honorable standing to physicians who did not designate themselves practitioners of an exclusive dogma or sectarian system, regardless of their educational backgrounds or actual practice.[11] To foster professional unity, the AMA authorized consultations and admission of all reputable practitioners into local societies. Some regular physicians believed the association of homeopaths with "men of high professional ideals" would turn them away from careers "begun in ignorance and innocence." Others were bolder in asserting that the best way to destroy homeopathy was to submerge it in orthodoxy.[12] Hugo R. Arndt, field secretary to the AIH in 1911, confirmed the success of this strategy in many states. On a trip through California, Utah, Colorado, South Dakota, North Dakota, Minnesota, Missouri, Illinois, and Ohio, he noted the success of the regulars' recruitment policy. Only twelve homeopaths remained in Utah, and an attempt to maintain a state homeopathic medical society had failed. In South Dakota, forty-five homeopaths had at one time maintained an active state society. However, gradually "our people have joined the 'regular' county societies, have been tendered official recognition on boards, and have wholly ceased to be aggressive in the advocacy of homoeopathic doctrines." Arndt noted that in some southern states, "our organizations are rapidly going to pieces," and that the homeopathic medical colleges in San Francisco and Detroit teetered on the brink of collapse due to lack of students.[13] In Minneapolis, many homeopaths, "young and old" joined old school societies although, according to Arndt, they maintained no loss of interest in homeopathy.[14]

Assessing their respective roles in the decline of their profession, homeopaths blamed each other as much as the "deliberate and farsighted policy of extinction, pursued systematically by the American Medical Association" for the "degeneration and demoralization" of their profession.[15] When the AIH redefined the meaning of homeopathy as a therapeutic specialty, speaker James Woods argued that the greatest barrier to its recognition by the "dominant school of medicine" were factors "inherent in Homoeopathy itself." The most salient of these factors was the literal interpretation of the *Organon* by Hahnemannians clinging to highly potentized drugs, the theory of dynamization, and the idea that a single dose of a remedy acted almost indefinitely. According to Wood, certain passages of the *Organon* "have done more to retard the growth of Homoeopathy than all other things combined." While judging it a "work of transcendent genius," he nevertheless argued that "we should take it for what it is worth and should not hesitate ruthlessly to reject that which experience, reason, and science declare absurd." "In short," he said, "we must be physicians first and Homoeopathists secondly—ever ready to utilize that which experience has demonstrated best for our patients."[16]

Homeopaths commonly referred to the period after 1900 as "homeopathy's dark ages."[17] Articles in medical journals during the first two decades of the twentieth century reflected a lack of confidence in homeopathy's ability to survive the dwindling enrollments in its schools and medical societies. Even the "once-splendid" Homoeopathic Medical Society of Chicago showed a decline in members. These disturbing trends, plus the deaths of older homeopaths who had actively supported the profession, resulted in a bleak picture for its future.[18] A homeopathic medical college was no longer a wise choice for those wishing to become doctors. The era of educational and professional reform stimulated by new scientific methods and knowledge as well as changing social norms was the beginning of the end of most homeopathic institutions, signaling the decline of women's professional and educational opportunities in American medicine. In the 1890s and into the first decade of the twentieth century, homeopathic schools in Boston, Chicago, Cleveland, Kansas City, Philadelphia (post-graduate school), and San Francisco appointed women to faculties. As schools and hospitals closed or dropped their affiliation with homeopathy, teaching opportunities and hospital staff appointments for women disappeared, as well.

In the 1870s and 1880s, leading medical schools (homeopathic and regular) elevated standards by lengthening courses, upgrading entrance and graduation requirements, and providing laboratory instruction. Homeopathic colleges were often in the forefront of such reforms. In 1891, the AIH required a four-year course of study in homeopathic schools for a college to receive accreditation by the national organization. By 1893, sixteen schools were accredited, with four still under review.[19] The most dramatic innovation of the nineties belonged, however, to Johns Hopkins Medical School (1892). With a full-time faculty chosen for its accomplishments in teaching and research, coeducational Johns Hopkins boasted a huge endowment, university affiliation, and a first-class teaching hospital.[20] Admission was highly selective, requiring college degrees of all entering students. Small class sizes, frequent testing, two years of instruction in the basic sciences, extensive laboratory work, and mandatory clinical instruction (clerkships) in internal medicine, surgery, obstetrics, and gynecology became the gold standard for a modern medical education. Many new subjects were added to the curriculum, including physiological chemistry, pharmacology, and bacteriology. Clinical teaching included all the traditional subjects along with new courses in dermatology, genito-urinary diseases, laryngology, psychiatry, pediatrics, ophthalmology, otology, and hygiene. The laboratory and clerkship replaced the lecture and demonstration as the best means of learning. Hospital work was an essential part of a Hopkins education. Taking patient histories, performing physical examinations, conducting routine laboratory tests, following patients' conditions, and suggesting methods of treatment were intimate parts of learning the "principles of practice."[21]

Although methods of curing disease did not advance apace with new diagnostic techniques identifying them, recent discoveries and the development of diagnostic technologies generated confidence in medicine's ability to develop cures. Although the stethoscope, ophthalmoscope, and laryngoscope had been used since the 1880s, physicians' ability to view evidence of disorder was enhanced in the 1890s by the introduction of the microscope, X-ray, chemical and bacteriological tests, along with machines such as the spirometer and electrocardiograph, which generated data on patients' physiological conditions. By 1905, laboratory tests could detect the organisms responsible for tuberculosis, cholera, typhoid, pneumonia, diphtheria, gonorrhea, and syphilis.[22] Microbiology improved upon the methods of Koch and Pasteur, aiding in the development of new vaccines against infectious diseases such as rabies, typhoid, cholera, and plague, as well as antitoxins to combat diphtheria and tetanus. These successes, along with increased emphasis on disease prevention, had a measurable impact on public health and people's confidence in the authority of science.

To remain competitive, homeopathic medical schools raised entrance requirements, lengthened their terms, and added new courses, laboratories, and clinical opportunities. Although a "thorough" and practical knowledge of homeopathic materia medica was still a stated goal of institutions; in practice, it was cast into the background as new, required courses were instituted. Many professors and students were not unhappy with the changes, believing that homeopathic therapeutics based on laborious and time-consuming methods of prescribing were behind the times.[23]

As public faith in the value of science increased and expert medical knowledge gained force as a "culturally compelling source of authority," the prestige of regular physicians increased along with lay deference, especially toward the specialized knowledge of academic physicians.[24] The replacement of staff physicians at Saint Louis Children's Hospital is a case in point. Founded in 1878 by Apolline Blair, member of a prominent Saint Louis family, the hospital was managed for several decades by local women connected by social status, friendship, and educational experiences; most had attended Mary Institute, an elite private girls' school in the city. In 1880, women managers staffed the hospital exclusively with homeopathic physicians with high social and professional standing in the community. Over the years, the homeopathic staff kept pace with advances in medical knowledge by modernizing patient care and establishing a pathology department for diagnostic testing. In 1905, commonly performed examinations included urinalysis, blood cultures for malaria and typhoid, throat cultures for diphtheria, evaluation of pus for gonococcus, and general postmortems. The 1907 annual report showed a 100 percent growth in numbers of patients treated from 1900 to 1907, photographs of immaculate new operating and surgical dressing rooms, increasing use of the dispensary, and an increase in diagnostic testing—from forty-seven per year in 1903 to 251 in 1907.[25]

But in 1910, concerned for the institution's status as well as its ability to provide up-to-date patient care, managers replaced the homeopaths with academic pediatric specialists; and in 1912, the hospital affiliated with Washington University. Robert Brookings, part of a new generation of millionaire businessmen, was instrumental in upgrading the debt-ridden medical school at Washington University, forging a new relationship between the hospital and college. President of the school's board of trustees in 1895, Brookings rallied influential and wealthy businessmen to support his efforts to transform the school on the Johns Hopkins model. In 1911, he negotiated the affiliation contracts between the reorganized medical school and its teaching hospitals.[26]

Events at Saint Louis Children's Hospital illustrate that wealthy businessmen considered scientific medical institutions especially worthy of philanthropy. Along with promoting scientific advancement, the institutions benefited people by providing better-trained doctors and improved patient care. Progressive, forward-looking philanthropists would not risk either their money or their reputations on enterprises with little chance of success. The decision of women managers in 1910 reflected popular opinion that homeopathic institutions were part of medicine's past rather than its future.[27] Declining enrollments in homeopathic medical schools support this conclusion.

Women's Medical Education

During the last decade of the nineteenth century, seven hundred women matriculated at nineteen of twenty-one homeopathic institutions, comprising 18 percent of all homeopathic graduates. Between 1900 and 1910, however, the number of women graduates dropped to less than half the previous decade, declining to 12 percent of all homeopathic graduates.[28] This corresponds to the roughly 50 percent reduction in numbers of women students at regular medical colleges.[29] Although six homeopathic schools closed or combined with other institutions during this ten-year period, sixteen schools most notable for significant numbers of women graduates remained.[30] Thus, lack of opportunity for homeopathic education does not explain the drop in women's attendance during this period, but rather a combination of factors: declining interest in homeopathy among medical students and the general public; increased duration and costs of a medical education; shifting patterns of women's careers and social values; and changes in the practice of medicine itself.

As Regina Morantz-Sanchez has argued, although the closing of women's medical colleges had a negative effect on female enrollments after 1900, it is likely that middle-class women found the study and practice of medicine less appealing, as well as less accessible than did previous generations of women. The twentieth-century emphasis on specialization and the identification of pathology in a specific function or body part, privileged the "science" over the "art" of medical practice.[31] New technological tools and procedures and "objective" forms of knowledge based on laboratory-controlled experiments devalued intuition, subjectivity, and the importance of contextualizing patients' lives. Pioneer women physicians like Elizabeth Blackwell criticized "radical objectivity" and scientific reductionism, associating it with a more masculine, less humane approach to patient care. At the same time fewer women entered medical schools, they swelled the ranks of social workers, teachers, and librarians, and became leaders in the rapid expansion of the nursing profession. Women were welcomed as osteopaths, naturopaths, chiropractors, and Christian Science healers, helping to popularize new and distinctive alternatives to mainstream medicine. Between 1890 and 1918, there were sharp increases in the number of women doing graduate work. And unlike the late nineteenth century when women who pursued education and professional careers rejected marriage, the proportion of professionals combining careers with marriage and children actually increased in the twentieth century. Nevertheless, balancing a medical career and family life became more difficult in the world of twentieth-century medicine. In order to be taken seriously and advance professionally, women had to demonstrate unreserved dedication to their work, often sacrificing personal social relationships.[32]

Perhaps the most significant factor in women's declining enrollments was the increased cost of a medical education. With the exception of schools affiliated with universities, the majority depended upon tuition income. New educational standards placed a heavy burden upon such institutions. As schools lengthened sessions, purchased expensive equipment, and upgraded facilities, costs were passed on to students. Although previous generations of women often received financial help from families to attend medical school, many had supported themselves and financed their education by working prior to entering school, as well as when school was not in session. When a medical education consisted of two or three years' of attendance during four or five-month sessions, this was a successful strategy. But when schools added preliminary requirements, lengthened training to four or more years and required eight or nine months' attendance, it was no longer viable. Elevated standards and higher tuition fees altered the economics of a medical education for women, putting it out of reach for many.[33]

The reduced attention to homeopathic materia medica and therapeutics in homeopathic schools, and an emphasis on the same subjects as those taught in regular schools provided no compelling reasons for choosing homeopathic colleges. Even the staunchest supporters of homeopathy agreed the curriculum required to prepare students to be modern physicians left little room for the study of homeopathic philosophy or therapeutics, believing postgraduate study offered the best means to that end. The vanishing distinctiveness of homeopathy, the acceptance of coeducation among many leading orthodox schools, and the overall decline of women medical students, contributed to the decreasing numbers of women homeopathic students.[34]

Homeopathic Colleges and Abraham Flexner

During the first decade of the twentieth century, the AMA's Council on Medical Education requested the Carnegie Foundation for the Advancement of Teaching to undertake a nationwide evaluation of medical schools. By the time Abraham Flexner's famous report, *Medical Education in the United States and Canada* (1910), appeared, student enrollment in homeopathic colleges had already declined from 1,909 at the turn of the century to 1,009.[35] Fifteen homeopathic colleges still existed at the time of Flexner's assessments. Those important for women students garnered mixed reviews. According to Flexner, the homeopathic medical school at Boston University had the highest entrance standards, with sixty out of sixty-two students entering with bachelor's degrees. Its laboratories were "unexcelled" in equipment and organization in respect to both research and teaching, and the school had access to adequate clinical material (patients). New York Medical College and Hospital for Women had "attractive" and "well kept" laboratories with simple but recent equipment, and the school possessed adequate clinical facilities and dispensary. Cleveland Homoeopathic Medical College had a "good" laboratory for physiology, but only fair provisions for teaching chemistry, anatomy, pathology, and bacteriology, with a poorly equipped dispensary and limited hospital clinical facilities. Hahnemann Medical College of Chicago fared less well. Flexner found its single laboratory in a "wretchedly dirty building" only "fairly equipped." There were no ward clinics in its adjoining hospital and only a fair dispensary. With the exception of the male-only New York homeopathic school, the homeopathic school at BU, and homeopathic departments at state universities, all depended primarily on student tuition to finance their institutions, making higher entrance standards or improved teaching, "distinctly unpromising."[36]

While Flexner's assessment of homeopathic schools was not altogether disparaging, he was adamant in asserting that the "ebbing vitality" and financial weakness of the homeopathic "sect" was the "logical outcome" of the "incompatibility of science and dogma." He included allopathy in his definition of medical sectarianism, claiming the "inevitability" of sects, prior to the placing of medicine on a scientific basis. "But now that allopathy has surrendered to modern medicine, is not homeopathy borne on the same current into the same harbor?" Reflecting the progressive view of the explanatory powers of modern science, Flexner wrote: "One cannot simultaneously assert science and dogma . . . science once embraced, will conquer the whole. Homeopathy has two options: one to withdraw into the isolation in which alone any peculiar tenet can maintain itself; the other to put that tenet into the melting pot . . . For everything of proved value in homeopathy belongs by right to scientific medicine and is at this moment incorporated in it; nothing else has any footing at all, whether it be of allopathic or homeopathic lineage."[37]

Although reforms in medical education had begun decades before Flexner's report, his work greatly accelerated the number of medical school closings (both homeopathic and regular) throughout the country.[38] The report was widely read, backed by the prestigious Carnegie Foundation, and influenced the medical profession, the public, and wealthy philanthropists in their ideas of what constituted a fully modern medical school. For example, although John D. Rockefeller was a patron of homeopathy throughout his life, the Rockefeller Foundation invested in the science and medicine of the future.[39] Flexner's ideal was modeled after Johns Hopkins—full-time faculty and research staff; extensive laboratory facilities for research in pathology, physiology, bacteriology, and pharmacology; extensive clinical teaching; small classes; and well-equipped medical museums and libraries. Unendowed schools lacking the financial resources to conform to the requirements began to close or merge with larger institutions.

Between 1900 and 1917, the number of homeopathic schools decreased from twenty-two to nine, and the number of students declined by two-thirds.[40] In 1918, New York Medical College for Women closed its doors. Its few remaining students transferred to New York Homoeopathic Medical College, which accepted women for the first time in its history. In that same year Boston University eliminated its homeopathic designation, responding to the widespread demands of alumni and students who believed survival of the medical school hinged on its identification with modern medical science.[41] Both schools had traditionally appointed women trustees, faculty, and hospital staff. But BU's commitment to women waned in its transformation into a regular institution. By 1919, there were no women among its forty-eight professors, and only six of forty lecturers were women.[42] Hahnemann Medical College in Chicago closed in 1922, as did the homeopathic medical department at Ohio State University—the longest surviving homeopathic medical department at a state institution.[43] By 1923, only two homeopathic institutions remained: the all-male Hahnemann Medical College of Philadelphia and New York Homoeopathic Medical College. Between 1910 and 1920, 129 women and 1,416 men graduated from homeopathic schools.[44] During the same period the number of women enrolled in regular colleges averaged about 550 per year with the total medical student population in the United States in 1920 at 13,798. In the next decade, homeopathic numbers dropped further with thirty women and 1,010 men graduating from homeopathic medical schools.[45] The population of homeopathic physicians was aging rapidly, and the medical system some had considered anachronistic even in the nineteenth century had, in all practicality, reached its intellectual and institutional end.

Homeopaths responded to the convergence of homeopathy and orthodoxy in a variety of ways. For some, homeopathic therapeutics became an incidental part (if any) of their medical practices. Giving up their homeopathic identities, they enthusiastically accepted invitations to join regular medical societies and discarded their "irregular" past. Others held joint membership in homeopathic and regular organizations. Although according to the AMA's new code of ethics, physicians wishing to join regular societies were prohibited from publicly identifying themselves as homeopaths, many continued to prescribe remedies based on symptom similarities.[46]

Vowing to prevent the disappearance of "true" homeopathy, leaders of the International Hahnemannian Association urged cooperation with the small minority in the AIH dedicated to the same goal. Still critical of the "loose unhomeopathic tendencies" of the AIH, leading Hahnemannians believed the best hope for homeopathy's survival lay in its members becoming active members of the parent organization.[47] Not everyone agreed, believing that cooperation and compromise would lead to the dissolution of homeopathy as they defined it. In 1892 Hahnemannian physicians founded Hering College of Homoeopathy in Chicago. As the location of two existing homeopathic schools, the city seemed an unlikely choice for yet another. Founders justified their decision to enter an already crowded field by their intention to provide a "radically different kind of teaching." Along with the fundamental branches of a medical education, including anatomy, chemistry, histology, physiology, microscopy, bacteriology, pathology, and surgery, Hering's chief objective was to teach and demonstrate "that pure homoeopathy is all that is necessary or desirable in the cure of the sick." Homeopathic philosophy—the "science and art" of healing as outlined in Hahnemann's *Organon of Medicine* and in *Chronic Diseases*—was taught by physicians who considered themselves "homoeopathists," first and "specialists" second.[48]

Hering attracted a respectable number of women students. Between 1892 and 1905 (the last date for which figures are available), fifty-three women graduated from the school. With the exception of Hahnemann Medical College of Chicago, it boasted the largest number of women graduates of any homeopathic school in the West during this period. Women regular physicians, hopeful that the increased acceptance of coeducation would result in proper recognition and professional opportunities for women, pointed to Hering's appointment of women faculty as an example of the progress women could and should expect to make. Signaling a rapprochement with their "irregular" sisters and a convergence of women's professional interests, the *Woman's Medical Journal* (a publication of women regulars) announced the appointments of homeopaths Carrie Shaw, chair of physiology and hygiene, and Mary Florence Taft, chair of the department of diseases of women.[49] Rhoda Pike-Barstow chaired Hering's all-female department of obstetrics, comprised of fellow homeopaths Margaret S. McNiff and Mary Van Alston

Maxon. Mary K. Mack joined the anatomical department in 1893.[50] The *Journal* further noted the election of Dr. Whitney, "a woman of culture and influence," to the Board of Trustees, and commended Hering for its "correct" representation of women.[51]

Yet when Abraham Flexner visited the school in April 1909, he found little to recommend it. According to his report, laboratory equipment was meager and clinical facilities "very limited." Students were not admitted to the hospital adjoining the college, and only a small dispensary allowed for clinical teaching.[52] Flexner included Hering among the six homeopathic colleges he deemed "utterly hopeless."[53] In 1895, three years after Hering was founded, faculty disputes resulted in the organization of yet another competing Chicago institution, Dunham Medical College, the aims and principles of which were almost identical to those of Hering. Dissatisfied that "noble materia medica, principles and philosophy" were crowded far to the background in many homeopathic colleges, Dunham announced its intent to "call back wanderers to the campfire, to revive and extend the grandest system of medicine ever given to the world."[54] Like Hering, Dunham appointed women to its faculty, including Anna Doven and Theresa K. Jennings. Rivalry between Hering and Dunham was "deplored by friends of homoeopathy," diminishing the strength of each and dividing the homeopathic community even further.[55] Dunham was in operation only seven years; relatively few students graduated, (fourteen women and fifty men) before its merger with Hering in 1902.

Unable to sustain several schools in one location, educators recognized the imperative of combining homeopathic resources; and in 1904, Chicago Homoeopathic Medical College merged with Hahnemann Medical College. Sometime after Flexner's 1909 assessment of Hering, that institution also became part of Hahnemann. One of the last surviving homeopathic colleges and the most important school for women's education in the western states, Hahnemann closed its doors in 1922.

Kentian Homeopathy

Advocates of Hahnemannian homeopathy also established the Post-Graduate School of Homoeopathics in Philadelphia in 1890. Funded largely by John Pitcairn Jr., the founder of Pittsburgh Plate Glass and a prominent member of the Swedenborg community in Bryn Athyn, Pennsylvania, the school based its teachings on the fifth edition of Hahnemann's *Organon* (1833), the last published before the founder's death.[56] James T. Kent, dean of the new school, was a former president of the IHA and editor of several homeopathic journals; today he is renowned as one of the most influential figures in the history of homeopathy, alongside Samuel Hahnemann and Constantine Hering. His major work, the *Repertory of the Homoeopathic Materia Medica* (1897), is still widely used, and according to one source, Kent's interpretation of Hahnemann's work "is the foundation for nearly every school and organization of homeopathy worldwide." To date, there is no comprehensive biography on Kent, and little information on his life. However, sources indicate that Kent became interested in the teachings of Emanuel Swedenborg through his association with John M. Scudder, owner and manager of the Eclectic Medical Institute of Cincinnati. Kent graduated in 1870 from the college where several members of the faculty, in addition to Scudder, were advocvates of Swedenborgianism.[57] In 1896, a student at the Post-Graduate School of Homoeopathics complained to a trustee that Kent had introduced the doctrines of Swedenborg into his teachings on homeopathy. Concerned that the school would develop a reputation for religious sectarianism, trustees investigated. Finding no corroborating proof, they considered the allegation simply one man's opinion, and the matter was dropped.[58]

For Kent, Hahnemann's doctrines were revelations of truth. But while Hahnemann described the vital force as an "automatic," nonmaterial "dynamis" that animates the material body, "spirit-like" in its essence, Kent's interpretation was more explicitly religious in orientation.[59] Kent's vital force was the "vice-regent of the soul," its "energy" proceeding from a supreme God, connecting the material with the spiritual worlds.[60] And as one Hahnemannian noted, "The identification of Hahnemann's vital force with the words 'spiritual,' or 'spirit-like,' though legitimate and illuminating, shocks the delicate sensibilities of the average scientist today . . . certain words . . . are 'taboo' in scientific circles."[61] Kent categorically rejected diagnoses based on pathological anatomy as the means of selecting homeopathic remedies. He promoted high-potency remedies, insisted on the validity of the concept of drug dynamization, and emphasized the paramount importance of mental symptoms in choosing remedies.[62] Believing mental symptoms indicative of the deepest levels of disturbances or illness, he developed patient "types" associated with particular drugs—"the ragged philosopher" in association with sulfur, for example.[63] Kent stressed Hahnemann's teachings that symptoms of mental "disorder" were key to discovering a correct remedy and to curing disease. "Man consists in what he thinks and what he loves . . . All medicines operate upon the will and understanding first . . . and ultimately upon the tissues, the functions, and sensations."[64] A free dispensary attached to the school opened on January 24, 1891. Acceptable clinical practices were limited to single doses of high-potency dynamized medicines, prohibiting the internal or external use of crude drugs.

Although his school lasted little more than ten years, in 1921 Kent's students and followers of his teachings were instrumental in organizing the American Foundation for Homeopathy to transmit the knowledge and practice of "real" homeopathy to a new (albeit limited) group of supporters in the twentieth century.[65] During the post-graduate school's history, thirty-eight physicians earned H.M. degrees (master of homeopathics); of those, nineteen were women. Five of the women received M.D. degrees from Woman's Medical College of Pennsylvania in the 1890s prior to entering the homeopathic post-graduate school.[66] Women were appointed as clinical assistants, lecturers, and professors; and in 1897, three of the six-member faculty were women: Fredericka E. Gladwin and S. Mary Ives, professors of paedology; and Julia Loos, professor of gynecology.[67]

The large percentage and role of women in these institutions also characterized the Society of Homoeopathicians. In 1896, thirty-nine members of the IHA founded a new organization pledging harmony with Hahnemann's *Organon of Medicine,* as interpreted by James Tyler Kent. Eleven of the founders were women, including five graduates from Kent's school. Recognizing Kent as "the foremost homoeopath in the world," eligibility for membership was restricted to his pupils, followers of his teaching (evidenced by four years' practice consistent with his philosophy), or four years' of "harmonious" associate membership in the organization. Julia Loos, coeditor with Kent of the society's journal, was a mainstay of the organization that spawned similar local groups dedicated to pure homeopathy. With little help from Kent during his last failing years, Loos edited and published the journal, personally shouldering much of the debt incurred. When Kent died in the spring of 1916, the journal ceased publication.[68]

Members of the Society of Homoeopathicians were considered extremists by the majority of homeopaths, who berated them for failing to see that "there may be good medical truth in other laws or principles than that enunciated by Hahnemann." According to one widely-read homeopathic medical journal: "To them the ordinary homeopath is a gross mortal, a mongrel physician, half allopath and half nothing, in no sense a true follower of Hahnemann. To them the International Hahnemannian is but one remove from his cruder colleague, deserving of a place alongside the allopath, the eclectic and the AIH. Fortunately there are not many of them."[69] At a time when homeopathic schools struggled for survival and homeopaths stressed homeopathy's compatibility with and similarities to modern medicine, the founding of strict homeopathic colleges and societies was a supreme embarrassment to the majority of homeopaths. Rather than consolidate efforts and resources to save those homeopathic schools with the most potential of meeting rising educational standards, many Hahnemannians withdrew their support, preferring the dissolution of what they called "mongrel" institutions. Although marginal to the broader homeopathic profession, orthodox Hahnemannians possessed a revolutionary zeal characteristic of the earliest generations of homeopaths in the United States. Their determination to magnify the differences between homeopathy and orthodox medicine separated them from the majority of their colleagues.

New York Hahnemannian Stuart Close attributed the loss of many homeopathic hospitals and most colleges to the failure of homeopaths to follow and teach the principles and technical methods of homeopathy's masters—Hahnemann, Boenninghausen, Hering, Lippe, Guernsey, Dunham, and Kent. Departure from their teachings, said Close has produced a failure in results: "Homeopathy has not failed, but its disloyal, badly taught, falsely professing practitioners have failed."[70] Some attributed the homeopathic demise to the increase in specialization and surgery in the homeopathic profession, as well as the declining emphasis on the therapeutics of homeopathy's general practitioners.[71] Universal disagreement as to what constituted homeopathic practice was cited by another, who lamented: "At present we are neither fish, flesh nor fowl, or even good red herring."[72] Others were more certain of their place in American medicine. As one professor succinctly put it: "We are physicians first, and homoeopaths afterward, and scientific men all the time."[73] From women's perspective, the last part of his statement was all too true.

Women Hahnemannians were a small minority of the homeopathic profession. In 1910, the IHA listed only thirty-four women members, compared with 309 in the AIH, yet their influence in preserving "pure" homeopathy exceeded their numbers.[74] Most of the women involved in the Society of Homoeopathicians were also leaders in the IHA. Julia Loos, Fredericka Gladwin, Julia Green, Margaret C. Lewis, Alice Bassett, and Florence Taft frequently presented papers, were bureau chairpersons, and members of the executive board.[75] And women's prominence in the IHA early in the twentieth century is reflected in the 1930 election of Grace Stevens as the organization's first woman president. The large role of women in the IHA is partly explained by the organization's small size and relatively large percentage of women compared with either the AIH or the homeopathic profession as a whole. Hahnemannians were also driven by something akin to a holy crusade—the determination to prevent "truths" of Hahnemann's homeopathy from dying out. But why were women especially active and even passionate in this cause? There was no bloodletting to protest as in the nineteenth century; no examples of egregious harm to women and children from the therapeutics of regulars to oppose. Although Hahnemannian institutions and organizations provided women with opportunities for teaching and leadership roles, career advancement alone does not explain their passion for a form of homeopathy most of their colleagues considered obsolete. Rather, dedication to an older, traditional version of homeopathy should be seen as a reaction not only against modern values of medical professionalism and practice but also against changes in American culture.

Hahnemannians and Antimodernism

Belief in the beneficence of material progress and the desire for the efficient control of nature, were fundamental precepts of modern progressive culture. American values were increasingly defined by external appearances, spiritual blandness, and material comfort. Urbanization, shaped by an interdependent marketplace, and the increasing bureaucracy of modern life, disturbed people's geographical roots and resulted in the fragmentation of individual identity, eroding the social and economic independence of the middle and upper classes. Liberal Protestantism lacked the moral intensity and absolutism of evangelical orthodoxy, leaving the faithful bereft of "moral truths" guiding individual and social behavior, contributing to a sense of weightlessness and spiritual void.[76] According to Jackson Lears, antimodern impulses recaptured an elusive "real life," instilled rigor, provided authentic experience, and restored a sense of selfhood as well as mystery to what some considered an over-civilized and inauthentic modernity. Individuals sought ways to prevent the resulting fragmentation of individual identity and autonomy, as well as restore spiritual meaning in everyday life.[77] Examples include the Arts and Crafts movement, which attempted to counteract both the culture of consumption and the disjunction of work and home brought about by industrial technology. Stressing the "simple life," and the ennobling power of work, advocates attempted to reunite "art and labor," by creating communities centered around small artisanal workshops.

Lears writes of the "hovering soul-sickness" of the late nineteenth century—a sense that life had become dry and passionless, lacking intensity of feeling. Believing that science had not explained the universe, some among the educated and affluent looked to the mystical and inexplicable to restore a sense of mystery and intense experience. Fin-de-siècle occultism, spiritual ecstasy, Oriental mysticism, along with secular therapies such as self-hypnosis and mind-cure, united individual identity with the cosmos, cultivating an awareness of one's dependence on the universe. Several in the "better educated strata" of antimodernists were advocates of Hahnemannian homeopathy, such as social reformer and Arts and Crafts advocate Mary Ware Dennett;

psychologist and philosopher William James; and poet Henry Wadsworth Longfellow.[78]

In Lears's opinion, antimodern dissenters were neither "cranks" nor part of the "late blooming flower" of the Romantic movement, but part of a leadership class "desperate to flee Victorian decorum and experience 'real life.'"[79] Rooted in reaction against secularizing tendencies, antimodernist expressions were a way of adapting to new and secular cultural modes through the "therapeutic ideal of self-fulfillment in *this* world through exuberant health and intense experience."[80]

Viewing Hahnemannian homeopathy as a thread of antimodern dissent in medicine shows the appeal it held for certain men and women. Hahnemann's "natural laws" offered absolutes, an external framework of "certainties" guiding physicians in curing the sick. At the same time, the metaphysical principle of a vital force gave spiritual meaning to sickness and health. The vagaries of microorganisms and physiology caused illness in some people, while others remained healthy even during epidemics. The role of the vital force explained all sickness, restoring individual accountability. Patients could meliorate hereditarian influences predisposing them to disease by employing homeopathic remedies along with proper exercise, diet, and other healthful practices. Over time, a vital force weakened by the crude drugs prescribed by allopaths could be revitalized with homeopathic remedies. Viewing the cause of illness as the result of a disturbed vital force—affecting mind, body, and spirit—advocates counteracted the fragmentation of individual identity by reinforcing traditional notions of the integral relationship of mind, body, and spirit in healing. Kentian homeopathy stressed a religious-like moral equation in health and sickness, whereby a morbid physical economy evidenced a disordered (and even evil) inner or mental state. For example, the exterior (physical body) of people who were insane or "evil" would reflect their inner mental illness or immorality. Mental disorder could develop from living on certain kinds of food which one found initially distasteful but continued to eat, believing one loved it. Thus, Kent interpreted Hahnemann's idea of psora (the fundamental cause of all contagious disease) not as an "itch vesicle" but as false consciousness or immorality.[81]

Professional values of Hahnemannians also provided a counterpoint to mainstream medicine, in which the "art" of medicine increasingly took a backseat to science. Authentication of diagnoses and prognoses of disease rested primarily on the outcomes of experiments in microbiological, physiological, and pharmacological laboratories. Modern physicians primarily defined disease as deviations from norms of measurable biological variables, diminishing the importance of social, psychological, and environmental influences. Divisions of medical disciplines into physiology, neurology, internal medicine, psychiatry, and psychology separated psychogenic from somatic factors. But although Hahnemannians opposed the reductionist and materialist orientation of scientific medicine, as well as that practiced by the majority of homeopaths, Kent's form of homeopathy was reductionistic in a different way. Kent believed physicians wasted their time searching for the causes of illness in people: "It is not the principal business of the physicians to be hunting in the rivers and the cellars and examining the food we eat for the cause of disease. The sick man will be made sick under every circumstance, whereas the healthy man could live in a lazaretto."[82] For Kent, homeopathic remedies alone restored and maintained health, hardly a mandate to reform the dangerous and unhealthy conditions existing in factories and tenements which contributed to people's mental and physical illnesses.

Although Hahnemannians denigrated the fragmentation and materialism of medical science, they used it to justify homeopathic claims to science, arguing that laboratory evidence revealed the power of minute substances to affect the human organism, and validated an unmeasureable, nonmaterial life force. Although homeopathy itself had not undergone demonstrable scientific testing, advocates believed the concept of infinitesimals was supported by new scientific discoveries. Recent knowledge of the miniscule diameter and weight of hydrogen molecules established a scientific basis for the power of infinitesimals.[83] They claimed the production of antitoxins confirmed Hahnemann's theory of dynamization and that homeopathy had been almost "out-dilutionized" by the process used in the manufacture of serums.[84] As Dr. Martha Boger of Portsmouth, New Hampshire, put it, homeopathy was "*ultra*-scientific!"[85] Hahnemannians argued that the practice of "real" homeopathy was more difficult—more intellectually rigorous—than regular or "mongrel" homeopathic medicine. Only a select few would become masters. According to Hahnemannian physician Ella Jennings, "It is a thousand times harder to be a good, true Homoeopathic prescriber like Hahnemann, Hering, Bayard, Lippe . . . than to practice the ordinary methods of the old school."[86]

As traditional symbols of professional status, such as hospital appointments and faculty positions, became unavailable to homeopaths and women, Hahnemannians developed an alternate status system, one equally accessible to both the sexes. Practitioners acquired professional status through stated commitment to Hahnemann's principles, active participation in Hahnemannian organizations, and reputations as "excellent" prescribers. While such reputations rested partly on successes claimed in case reports presented at professional meetings, they were also evidenced by the number of dedicated patients who supported their practices. Turning to patients for support, Hahnemannian practitioners organized local clubs to educate patients on what to expect from a "real" homeopath, encouraging them to assess individual physicians according to specific criteria. The Boenninghausen Club of Boston published a pamphlet in 1900 designed to help people determine whether they were being treated by a "follower of Hahnemann" or by "one who merely lays claim to that honor without comprehending its meaning."[87] The list of prohibited practices included all local applications—including douches, salves, and gargles—which, according to the publication, either caused injury or so modified symptoms that the task of selecting the correct remedy proved impossible. Morphine or other sleep- or pain-relieving drugs retarded recovery and concealed important symptoms. The pamphlet informed readers that no emetics, purgatives, patent medicines, heart stimulants, or coal tar products would be found among the remedies of Hahnemannians, whose concern for patients' comfort was expressed in a search for genuine cure rather than palliation. The document stressed that homeopathy, founded on "natural law," could not fail. Physicians might not find the proper remedy, patients might not provide accurate accounts of their symptoms, or the diseased body might not respond to treatment, but having withstood the crucial test of time and experience, homeopathy could not fail.[88]

In some ways the Hahnemannians' critique of mainstream medicine was similar to that of an earlier generation of women regular physicians who criticized the radical objectivity and scientific reductionism of modern medicine. Women pioneers like Elizabeth Blackwell believed "objectivity" and the laboratory medicine that promoted it would lead to the objectification of patients and a less humane, holistic approach to patient care. According to Blackwell, preoccupation with the laboratory lessened the importance of physicians' skills in clinical observation and "character" at the bedside, threatening the doctor/patient relationship. But Blackwell's critique of modern medicine was deeply influenced by her conceptions of gender and framed in the language of domesticity. She associated empathic and relational qualities with the "female," counterposing them to the science of the laboratory, identifying it with male objectivity.[89] Although such "feminine" attributes were considered essential to the success of homeopathy, women Hahnemannians did not "engender" homeopathic practice. Intuition, circumspection and tact, patience in observing and listening, and knowledge of the human heart were essential qualities for all Hahnemannians. Like older male regular physicians who opposed the new professionalism, Hahnemannians framed their argument against modern medicine as a preservation of an older, more holistic style of professional behavior—one accessible to both males and females.

Chapter 7 | **Struggle for Survival, 1920–1930**

RECALLING HER EXPERIENCES with homeopathy during the early decades of the twentieth century, longtime advocate Elinore Peebles (1897–1992) said, "The trouble with us in New England was that we were used to good homeopaths, and good homeopathic prescribing, and we weren't about to accept a doctor who practiced with homeopathic pills in one pocket and antibiotics in the other."[1] Raised in Newtonville, Massachusetts, by a Swedenborgian mother and a father who was a homeopathic physician, Peebles devoted much of her ninety-five years to the preservation of Kentian homeopathy, which she described as a mixture of Hahnemannian and Swedenborgian philosophy. She felt keenly the loss of homeopathy's status, as well as the decline and dissolution of its once vibrant institutions.

By 1923, all but two homeopathic medical schools had eliminated their homeopathic designations or closed their doors. Leaders waged largely unsuccessful battles to retain control of homeopathic hospitals, and homeopathic medical societies languished for lack of enthusiastic young physicians.[2] Yet interest in homeopathy among patients and physicians did not disappear along with its institutions. According to Peebles, homeopathic patients "truly . . . suffered. They did not want to go to any other kind of doctor, but they had no choice." Although patients took care of themselves as much as possible, she said, at least in New England, "they all continued to work for homeopathy."[3] Despite a general pessimism that pervaded the homeopathic profession during this time, some advocates expressed cautious optimism that somehow homeopathy would prevail and even be scientifically confirmed by new discoveries in immunology and physics. However, during this period of institutional decline, intraprofessional relations deteriorated to their lowest point.

132

The lessening of antagonism between homeopaths and regulars that brought about their professional cooperation had been more easily accomplished than cooperation *among* homeopaths, including doctors and patients. The increasing influence of lay advocates is reflected in Peebles's description of the reception given to homeopathic physician Ursula Webber upon her arrival in Boston.

According to Peebles, Webber "did a beautiful job" selling herself to the local homeopathic community. But, "she turned out to be a real disaster, and we were delighted when she moved on. You see, you couldn't fool these New England homeopaths—they knew a good homeopathic doctor when they saw one."[4] Decades later, homeopathic physician Richard Moskowitz noted the power and influence of Boston's lay advocates when he moved to the city in 1982. Although he had planned a short sabbatical before establishing his medical practice, Peebles sought him out within a few days of his arrival. Quizzed on his knowledge of Hahnemann and Kent, Peebles and "The Boston Ladies" scrutinized his ability to practice "true" homeopathy. Finding him acceptable and "in a voice that brooked no contradiction," Peebles told the young doctor that "there hadn't been a homeopath in Boston for twenty-five years, and that I'd better get busy."[5]

While lay advocates such as Elinore Peebles played a significant role in homeopathy's survival early in the twentieth century as well as it's rebirth in later decades, disputes among laypeople and physicians alike over who deserved to be called a "real" homeopath had a corrosive effect on the profession. And although homeopaths blamed the AMA's efforts at educational reforms for unacceptable ratings of most homeopathic colleges, they also blamed themselves for the low state of their profession.

General practitioners felt the increase in specialization, especially surgery, accounted for the demise of homeopathic prescribing.[6] Others criticized homeopaths' lack of support for their own institutions. Citing the decision of Iowa's state legislature to cut appropriations to state schools in 1923, including funding for the department of homeopathic materia medica and therapeutics, an editorialist noted that many homeopaths in the state, some of whom were state officials, sent their sons to "old school" medical colleges.[7] And, Hahnemannian homeopaths allowed homeopathic colleges to close, rather than support those they believed perverted Hahnemann's teachings. Others believed the failure of homeopathic organizations and institutions was the direct result of professional and personal jealousy among homeopathic physicians, as well as their general lack of organizational, management, and business skills.[8] Adherents of both the high-potency philosophy (Hahnemannians) and the low-potency approach (progressives) blamed each other for the crisis.

Some members of the AIH and IHA argued in favor of unifying the two national homeopathic organizations to create a system of federated medical societies similar to that of the AMA, but members could not agree on common goals and purposes.[9] Although many homeopaths held joint membership in the two organizations, inflammatory rhetoric over the issue of high- or low-potency prescribing continued unabated—reflecting different understandings of science, practice, and professionalism. At an AIH meeting in 1924, one impatient physician sounded a familiar but unheeded appeal: "Let us stop calling each other names and all work together to bring a state of cohesion [to the profession]."[10] Why, how, and with what success women worked toward this end is an important aspect of the subject.

Women in the American Institute of Homoeopathy

Although the number of women entering the homeopathic profession declined drastically after 1910, women homeopathic physicians and patients were especially active in efforts to ensure continued opportunity for women's medical education. Laywomen and female physicians affiliated with the American Institute of Homoeopathy funded scholarships for worthy female medical school candidates, formed local and national women's leagues, and promoted homeopathic education.

In several cities, laywomen maintained more of a "sense of purpose" and organization on behalf of homeopathic medicine than did homeopathic physicians.[11] For example in Detroit, Mrs. R. Milton Richards, whose husband was a homeopath, presided over the Ladies' Homeopathic Student Loan Association.[12] Lester E. Siemon, president of the AIH in 1924, commended the excellent work of Mrs. Caron, a member of the loan association, who successfully appealed to the AIH for donations. Inspired by Caron's enthusiasm and dedication to the homeopathic cause, Siemon stated his determination to "make use" of connections with other women's organizations throughout the country.[13] In 1911, AIH field secretary Dr. Hugo R. Arndt expressed his enthusiasm over the large attendance at a recent meeting of the "ladies" Homoeopathic League in Saint Paul, Minnesota. Organized "some time ago," Arndt told his colleagues that "people . . . have forgotten the great things done in former times by similar organizations . . . Women have a way of doing some kinds of work, as propagandistic work, far more effectively than we men do, and we should be more eager to utilize their helpful ability."[14]

Although it is unclear when the Women's National Homoeopathic League was founded, women in various cities organized local leagues affiliated with the national organization for both social and educational purposes. For

example, at the 1910 meeting of the American Institute, the Woman's Homoeopathic League of Minnesota reported good attendance at "parlor lectures" on
the "History of Medicine" and "dietetics," as well as meetings where women
discussed the status of homeopathic medical education at the University of
Minnesota.[15] In 1924, the wife of Saint Paul homeopath E. L. Mann, was
elected president of the national organization, whose annual meetings were
held in conjunction with those of the American Institute. While calling
themselves a "social organization of the homemakers of the medical profession," the women were aware of the important past contributions laywomen
had made to homeopathic institutions. As Mann noted in her May 1924
report, "Women have always been credited with being money getters and in
the last generation have also shown their ability as money makers."[16] Mann
urged women to extend the number of local leagues intended to raise scholarship funds by drumming up enthusiasm among women interested in homeopathy in their communities. "Form a League, hold meetings . . . do fancy work,
have a sale . . . get some of the local Doctors to talk to you on the needs
of homoeopaths, study dietetics, home nursing—emergencies . . . get
acquainted, work together and make the meetings enjoyable as well as prof-
itable [through] cards! lunches! *Ma* Jong parties!" Mann reminded women
that moneymaking was a "ladies' game . . . there is no *Pa* Jong."[17] In August
1924, the Women's National Homoeopathic League added $1,311 to its
scholarship fund with contributions from leagues in Minnesota, Rhode Island,
Ohio, and Michigan. While funds were available to both male and female students, the women's attention seemed focused more toward aiding their over-
worked physician husbands by educating "young needy men" to lighten the
load and share the burden of "our husband Doctors."[18]

The agenda of the Institute Fraternity of the AIH, however, focused on
helping women with the costs of a twentieth-century medical education.
Organized in 1905 to encourage the participation of women homeopathic
physicians in the AIH as well as for social and collegial purposes, the fraternity gradually narrowed its focus. In 1918 it established a scholarship loan
fund along with three memorial funds, and between 1918 and 1925, offered
seven women students financial aid. Candidates were required to have a college degree, and be ethical, talented, and "more capable than the average" to
be an asset to the fund.[19] According to the fraternity's literature, every woman
received training in "homoeotherapy."[20] In 1927 the Institute Fraternity was
incorporated as the Women's Homoeopathic Medical Fraternity. Members
believed the new name more accurately reflected their principal objective—
educating women as homeopathic physicians.[21] Homeopath Mary E. Hanks of
Chicago, a longtime member and treasurer of the Institute Fraternity in 1924,

estimated the loan fund had accumulated around $20,000 by 1927 and loaned approximately $1,500 yearly. In Hanks's opinion, if the fraternity could "keep shoving a few good women into the profession constantly, it will help keep homoeopathy alive."[22]

But the survival of homeopathic knowledge and practice depended upon more than a "few good women." The profession was divided by ideology, partisanship, competition for funds to aid remaining homeopathic institutions, and different methods of assimilating into the medical mainstream. Any attempts to unify homeopaths behind a single set of goals to preserve homeopathy would need to take into account the various meanings of homeopathy to individual practitioners, to what extent they identified themselves as homeopaths, either to themselves or others, and their various methods of assimilation. While the process varied, most homeopaths did not jettison every aspect of their homeopathic training, knowledge, and identity, and simply disappear into the ranks of orthodoxy. Some homeopaths retained membership in homeopathic organizations and continued to prescribe homeopathically, yet did not publicly identify themselves as homeopaths.[23] Joint memberships in homeopathic and regular medical societies were not uncommon. For example, Chicago homeopaths Mary E. Hanks and Julia Strawn were simultaneously members of the AMA, the AIH, and the Chicago Homoeopathic Medical Society. Conrad Wesselhoeft (1884–1962), prominent Boston homeopath and 1911 graduate of Harvard Medical School, took pride in his membership in the Massachusetts Medical Society and valued his association with many "ambitious open-minded allopaths . . . [finding them] eager to know more about what Homoeopathy could do."[24]

In certain circumstances, homeopathic physicians did not emphasize or explain their homeopathic leanings to patients. For example, when patients seemed unaware of the distinctions between homeopathy and regular medicine, physicians simply would not make a point of mentioning their affiliation with homeopathic medicine.[25] According to Margaret C. Lewis, a graduate of Woman's Medical College of Pennsylvania in 1895 and Kent's post-graduate school in 1897, most patients appreciated individual doctors but not homeopathy in general.[26] Homeopath Cornelia Chase Brant of New York City agreed, believing the average layperson chiefly wanted relief from pain or discomfort, and did not care whether the doctor was homeopathic.[27] Homeopath Morris Elting Gore of Orange, New Jersey, found patients "quite ignorant and indifferent." Gore believed the "last thing" his patients desired was to be educated on the subject of homeopathy—"all they want is a prescription and a cure in short order."[28] Baltimore's Alice Parkhurst, a homeopathic practitioner for forty years, believed her exterior sign, "Homeopathic Physician," confused patients who did not know the meaning of homeopathy. In her opinion, her mostly female patients came to her because she was a woman physician.[29] And although individual homeopaths may have practiced according to homeopathic principles, whether they acknowledged this in conversations with regular physicians and patients depended on the particular circumstances and personalities involved, and the professional risks of such revelations.

Connecticut homeopath Stella Root enjoyed "cooperative" experiences with "old school" doctors with whom she "made no emphasis" of her homeopathic leanings.[30] Yet homeopath Elizabeth Wright was appointed attending physician at New England Hospital for Women and Children with full knowledge on the part of hospital officials that she would practice strict Hahnemannian or "pure" homeopathy there. In the opinion of Boston homeopath Mary R. Lakeman, Wright's acceptance at the hospital reinforced her own belief that female doctors were less prejudiced toward homeopaths than male physicians.[31] Despite the blending of homeopathy with mainstream medicine, many homeopaths, including progressives, maintained their identification with the homeopathic school (as they understood it) through membership in the AIH and local homeopathic societies. Most were eager to keep homeopathy alive in some form. With their institutional power gone, homeopaths in both factions turned to their patients for help.

In the era of "foundation building" where "men of great wealth" endowed scientific and educational institutions, members of both the IHA and AIH discussed targeting wealthy homeopathic patients to support the few remaining homeopathic institutions.[32] But only the newly organized American Foundation for Homoeopathy (AFH) presented a comprehensive (albeit overly-ambitious) plan of research, education, and promotion involving laypeople as well as doctors in the preservation of homeopathy. While different interpretations of homeopathy had historically divided homeopaths, founders of the AFH believed conducting modern scientific research into homeopathy would eliminate arguments based on subjective experience and abstract theory, thus uniting them under a mantle of science, which would justify the truth and efficacy of traditional (Hahnemannian) homeopathic philosophy and practice.

Women of the American Foundation for Homoeopathy

In 1920, IHA members Julia Loos and Julia Green interested ten homeopathic physicians in a plan to preserve "pure homeopathy." Although they rejected incendiary "high-" and "low-potency" rhetoric, promoting nonpartisanship instead, most were followers of James Tyler Kent and dedicated to the traditional philosophies and therapeutics of Samuel Hahnemann. On June

28, 1924, the organization incorporated as the American Foundation for Homoeopathy. Trustees included three female and four male physicians and one layman.[33]

With an office in Washington, D.C., Loos and Green established the structure of the new organization, consisting of four bureaus—publicity, research, publication, and education. Goals included the establishment of a major research center and hospital, a post-graduate school, and the development of lay leagues throughout the country. Julia Green envisioned a major research center in the capital where investigation of clinical cases and "proving," laboratory tests, and scientifically controlled studies would correlate physics and chemistry with homeopathy, placing it "where it belongs in the scientific world."[34]

The AFH corresponded to an older model of homeopathic professional organizations ,where women physicians were frequently elected to leadership positions and laywomen were the driving force behind fund-raising activities.[35] Women were founders, members of the board of trustees, and teachers in the post-graduate school. The seven physician trustees also reflected the aging of the homeopathic profession. At age fifty-three, Julia Green was the youngest trustee.

Recognizing women's diminished status within the broader arena of American medicine, Green worried that the Foundation's progress would be hindered by close identification with women. She wrote the trustees: "I have an idea that some interested physicians and laymen would have more faith in the work we have undertaken if the leader were a man," suggesting they might want a male chairman.[36] But either because they thought her concerns unfounded or because they believed no one would work as hard on the Foundation's behalf, Green became the first permanent chairman of the board of trustees in 1923.[37]

Although many Hahnemannians valued and admired Julia Loos for her knowledge of homeopathic philosophy, materia medica, as well as her complete dedication to the "cause," Loos's personality was considered "difficult." One candid obituary noted: "No one doubted her loyalty to homoeopathy, her integrity, her earnestness, but to some . . . she seemed changeable, inarticulate, more or less impossible."[38] As cofounder of the radical Homoeopathician Society and editor of its journal, Loos was well known for her dogmatic high-potency advocacy.[39] Julia Green, on the other hand, was universally admired and respected even by those considering Hahnemannians "high-potency cranks."[40] In a profession where personality conflicts fueled ideological divisions, Julia Green was the AFH's greatest asset. Politically astute, with a keen sense of humor and contagious enthusiasm, Green was a popular leader in the Foundation's efforts to pull together a fractious profession.

Green's choice of a homeopathic medical school was made in the last decade of the nineteenth century, reflecting the combined influences of family tradition as well as reforms in medical education that raised admission standards. Born in Malden, Massachusetts, into an upper-middle-class New England family, she was six years old when her family moved to Washington, D.C. Green was grateful to her parents for providing the means for two college degrees. After graduating from Wellesley College in 1893, Green's desire to help people and serve a social purpose prompted her decision to study medicine.[41] Although she considered applying to Johns Hopkins, only forty miles from her home, Green believed her science grades from Wellesley were not high enough to ensure admission. Having been under homeopathic treatment throughout her life, she read books on homeopathic philosophy, eventually deciding to attend the "best" homeopathic college. After graduating second in her class in 1898 from Boston University School of Medicine and completing an internship at Memorial Hospital for Women and Children in Brooklyn, N.Y., Green established a medical practice in Washington, D.C. in 1900. Active in the suffrage movement and a variety of professional and civic organizations in the capital, Green was a modern-day Clemence Lozier, often holding informal talks and lectures in her home for patients interested in learning more about homeopathy.[42] Her belief that patients educated in homeopathic theory and therapeutic principles would create demand for Hahnemannian physicians became the underlying premise of the Foundation's goals.

Green considered the establishment of lay leagues a high priority. Possibly influenced by similar leagues in Germany, she helped establish the first layman's league affiliated with the AFH in Washington, D.C. on December 6, 1924.[43] Comprised mostly of Green's female patients, members typically had some experience with homeopathic treatment and were eager to learn more about it. By December 1925, the league had sixty-two members.[44] At a time when many physicians distanced themselves from patients, and medical knowledge was viewed as increasingly complex, comprehensible only to medically trained physicians, lay leagues offered patients the opportunity for partnership with physicians. Doctors attended monthly meetings, presented lectures, answered member's questions, and encouraged patients to become knowledgeable about homeopathic philosophy and therapeutics. League membership empowered patients, enabling them to assess individual practitioners according to specific criteria, placing themselves and their families under the care of doctors whose practices were consistent with them.

By the spring of 1925, Green believed the foundation needed a full-time field worker to publicize its work and raise funds. Although we do not know when Green and Mary Ware Dennett first became acquainted, trustees requested that Green sound out Dennett on the proposition of becoming the Foundation's special field representative. Green reported back that Dennett "is intensely interested in Homoeopathy and in the foundation plan and states that she has been successful in the past in raising funds by the indirect method," by arousing people's enthusiasm for a cause so that they gave money to it.[45] Dennett's personal history and ideology as well as her role in the AFH, reveal the complex influences of gender, generation, intraprofessional politics, professional aspirations, family tradition, and the changing concepts of homeopathy and feminism among patients and physicians during the early decades of the twentieth century.

Mary Ware Dennett—Special Representative to the AFH

Honed through years of involvement in progressive reform activities such as the Twilight Sleep movement, single tax, international free trade, the Woman's Peace Party, and the League for Progressive Democracy, Dennett possessed superior organizational and political skills. As a new board member of the National American Woman's Suffrage Association in 1910, Dennett quickly earned a reputation for diplomacy by "appeasing all egos while maintaining strict neutrality" in an organization plagued by factionalism.[46] In 1915 Dennett organized the first birth-control organization in the country, the National Birth Control League. Unlike Margaret Sanger, whose efforts to secure birth control for women were directed at circumventing obscenity laws by placing information and devices in the hands of physicians for distribution, Dennett fought for complete repeal of the Comstock antiobscenity laws, arguing women had a *legal* right to such services.[47]

Dennett's attraction to homeopathic medicine stemmed partly from a family tradition of homeopathic care.[48] Born into an upper-middle-class Boston family, both Dennett's mother and sister Clara were ardent homeopathic patients; and her uncle, Carleton Spencer, was a prominent homeopathic practitioner and educator in New York City.[49] But Dennett's advocacy of homeopathy also was connected to her ideas on women's rights; individual freedom; the intimate relationship between science, art, and religion; and formed part of a broader cultural critique of early-twentieth-century industrialized society. Dennett considered herself an insurgent, part of the vanguard of social radicalism. She argued for the erotic rights of women, including birth control, subscribed to *The Masses*, and was a member of Heterodoxy—a group of radical feminists who met regularly to debate social issues such as free love, divorce, collective child rearing, and anarchy.[50] A leader in Boston's Arts and Crafts Movement, Dennett considered "all special privileges" the craftsmen's enemy, including monopolies and trusts, corrupt legislatures, and a "weighty" military establishment. In her view, reunification of art and labor in the work-place would eliminate the "shoddy" commodities produced in America's industrial workplace. But more importantly, it would counteract the degrada-tion and exploitation of workers, reintegrating the creative (or spiritual) and intellectual elements of human nature with one's work. In her ideas of labor, like those on human sexuality and medicine, Dennett combined physical, intellectual, and spiritual purposes.[51]

In 1919 Dennett published a pamphlet, *"The Sex Side of Life": An Expla-nation for Young People*, demystifying and explaining the physiology of sex, including controversial topics such as masturbation, venereal disease, and birth control.[52] In 1921, actively involved in testing the Comstock antiob-scenity laws, which prohibited the distribution of birth control information through the United States Postal Service, Dennett met with Dr. Hubert Work, former president of the AMA and assistant postmaster general. Work announced he was "opposed to the entire subject [birth control]," arguing that Dennett seemed to want to "instruct everybody how to have illicit intercourse without the danger of pregnancy."[53] The following year, Work rose to the posi-tion of postmaster general, and instructed post offices throughout the country to post bulletins announcing that sending or receiving material pertaining to birth control would be considered a criminal act.[54]

Deeply suspicious of organized medicine, Dennett believed people's free-dom to choose health practitioners, like their freedom to make personal deci-sions regarding sexuality and reproduction, was threatened by the increasing bureaucracy of modern society—especially the political power of organized medicine, which she termed a "growing medical monopoly."[55] She resented the "tyranny of experts" who undermined the reasoned opinions and common sense of individuals holding different views. Her attraction to antimodern impulses such as traditional homeopathy and Arts and Crafts, were responses to the growing depersonalization and segmentation of a modern, industrial-ized society. Although Dennett never used the term "holistic" to describe her conceptions of the body, homeopathy's "natural laws" and its concept of a spirit-like "vital force" connecting the mind, body, and spirit corresponded to Dennett's ideal of fully integrated individuals.[56] She likened the homeopathic practitioner to an artist. The homeopath's "little dose" like the artist's "great stroke" seems small in relation to their final results; yet "effort of a lifetime . . . lies behind that little single act."[57] And although she rejected institutionalized religion and disparaged homeopaths who treated homeopathy like a church or a creed "instead of like a science and a demonstrable art,"[58] Dennett viewed herself as a "decidedly more religious person" than when "under the thralldom (sic) of conventional Christianity."[59] For her, homeopathy was a kind of secularized religion, "part of the plan of the universe, of what it means to help work out natural laws and not hinder them."[60]

Recent scholarship shows that between 1920 and 1950 holistic trends both within and outside of mainstream medicine were influenced by peoples' perceptions that modern life was increasingly dominated by technology, bureaucracy, and commercial relations. Intense condemnation of reductionism in medicine, dominated by laboratory research and technology, fueled the popularity of medical alternatives, such as homeopathy, naturopathy, and holism, within mainstream medicine.[61] But Dennett's advocacy of Hahnemannian homeopathy was not simply an antimodern impulse driven by nostalgia. She criticized homeopaths that prescribed solely on the "old dictum" that diseases show themselves by symptoms, believing diseased states or tendencies exist prior to any "ordinarily detectable symptoms."[62] According to Dennett, physicians who based treatment solely on symptoms missed important opportunities to "create and conserve" health. Her continued dedication to homeopathy was fueled by her belief that modern science would provide the means for accurate diagnoses, selection of remedies, and proper potencies. With its ambitious plan for research and clinical studies, the Foundation seemed the very vanguard of homeopathic progress.[63] Its emphasis on patient and physician education as well as its promotion of an equal role for laypeople (including her prominent role as lay "expert") appealed to Dennett's sense of egalitarianism. But concerned that trustees would consider her work with the birth control movement controversial—a hindrance to the promotion of homeopathy—Dennett offered to withdraw herself from consideration for the position.[64]

Julia Green assured her the board "would not hesitate in the least having Dennett connected with the Foundation." One male trustee suggested she would be an asset.[65] Indeed, during one of Dennett's first official speaking engagements, a joint convention of the AIH and IHA, she was asked to comment on a paper dealing with birth control. Many physicians asked her to suggest books on the subject, and wanted to know the "best authorities" on birth control methods. Afterward, she wrote to Julia Green: "Again I feel funny to have the professionals turn to a layman for information!"[66] Dennett's comment was disingenuous, for she had great experience in the role of "lay expert" in both the twilight sleep and birth control movements. It was precisely the role she undertook as special lay representative to the AFH.

From the beginning of her tenure with the AFH, Dennett reminded Green that she was not a professional fund-raiser—not a "forthright money beggar"—but that she would promote the organization and meet with interested people, "which should produce money."[67] Julia Green told Dennett that the campaign would be left "squarely in her hands." Throughout Dennett's two and a half years with the AFH, they corresponded almost daily. Green was a constant consultant and booster, following up on Dennett's visits to doctors and patients with written appeals for donations. They discussed Dennett's best approach to people based on their personalities, past behavior, or local politics among homeopaths. Dennett began working from her home in New York City in October 1925. From then to September 1927, she met with homeopathic doctors and patients in New England, New York, Maryland, Pennsylvania, and the Midwest. Her richly detailed reports to Green illuminate peoples' perceptions of the status of the homeopathic profession, details of women's medical practices and professional relationships, and the various meanings of homeopathy to patients.

Physicians in the northeastern states held little hope for homeopathy's future. Doctors in New York City complained of uninterested patients, many recent immigrants, who simply wanted relief from pain or discomfort, not caring whether the doctor was homeopathic.[68] Some male physicians active in the AIH opposed the Foundation's premise that laypersons had a role equal to physicians in the preservation of homeopathy, or that the impetus should come from outside the AIH. New York homeopath Frederick M. Dearborn told Dennett: "I am an organization man, a former president of the American Institute, and I have no patience with anything which disrupts the organization . . . if anything is done for homeopathy it should be done through the organization [the AIH]."[69]

Dennett's reports show that the majority of male homeopaths in New York City, although discouraged about the state of their profession, were interested in the Foundation's program. New York's women homeopaths, however, were unusually antagonistic, believing the AFH was in some way associated with the previously all-male New York Homoeopathic Medical College. After several women physicians refused to see her, Dennett learned that women homeopaths in New York had recently been involved in a bitter court case with the men's homeopathic college. According to Dr. Rita Dunlevy, the women believed their medical college had been "wrested" from their control by leading male homeopaths who wanted to "'wreck their work and control their property.'" Dr. Gertrude Mack flatly refused to see Dennett, believing the AFH was connected in some way to New York Homoeopathic Medical College. Mack told Dennett she was "sorry" for her to be "turned loose in this city . . . You won't get one bit of sympathy from any of the women, I assure you."[70] In a letter to Green, Dennett wrote that although none of the defendants in the case had anything do to with the AFH, trustee Alonzo Austin was apparently "on friendly terms" with an individual defendant of the men's college.[71] Speaking by telephone with Dennett, Mack said: "The whole profession had left the few women in New York to fight their battle alone, had absolutely gone back on them." According to Dennett, Mack would have nothing to do with anything homeopathic "no matter what it might be."[72]

In other cities, Dennett's reputation as a social reformer and women's rights activist opened doors. She was greeted with enthusiasm by an earlier generation of women homeopaths who considered her a sister in shared battles for women's rights, suffrage, and other progressive reforms. Dennett found Dr. Alice Butler of Cleveland "overwhelmingly cordial to me personally." Although Dennett was not aware that Butler was a homeopath, for many years the two attended the same conventions and served together on committees. In her report to Green, Dennett wrote that it was "hard to say whether her [Butler's] enthusiasm is for the idea [of the Foundation] or for the person who presents it."[73] Dr. Jennie Medley, one of Philadelphia's pioneer women homeopaths, received Dennett with "open arms" when she learned she was the same Mrs. Dennett who used to be secretary of the National American Woman Suffrage Association.[74] Dennett was also "delightfully welcomed" by Boston homeopaths Fredericka Moore, Susan M. Coffin, and Mary R. Lakeman, who knew Dennett from her work in sex education. Employed by the Department of Public Health, all three used Dennett's pamphlet, *The Sex Side of Life*, in their work with adolescents. The physicians were especially interested in knowing of any Foundation plans for preventive work among children.[75]

Although Boston physicians generally believed their patients were knowledgeable about homeopathy and potentially interested in the Foundation, New England homeopaths were the most pessimistic regarding homeopathy's future. In 1918, with enrollments declining and alumni and faculty urging changes, the homeopathic medical school at Boston University became an orthodox institution while continuing, for a time, to offer courses in homeopathy.[76] Although Boston homeopath Alice Bassett subsequently agreed to teach in the Foundation's post-graduate school, Dennett's first meeting with her was less than auspicious. Bassett believed it "useless" to try to save homeopathy, either as a name or as a school, especially in Boston. As a professor at Boston University Medical School, Bassett said she was disheartened by the "aggressive prejudice and antagonism" of many of her medical students "scared to death of the tag "homoeopathy," objecting to having it "stuffed down their throats." Recently, four of her students had "backed out" because another well-meaning homeopathic physician had "undertaken to whoop up homeopathy to them."[77]

In the 1920s, Boston's homeopaths were also engaged in a battle to retain Massachusetts Homoeopathic Hospital. As Ronald Numbers and other scholars have shown, New England's powerful phalanx of Christian Science, mental science, new thought, and psychotherapy offered more distinct psychologically and spiritually oriented alternatives to mainstream medicine than homeopathy.[78] According to Boston homeopath Benjamin Woodbury, the ranks of the "drugless cults" swelled not because they cured more people, but because the metaphysical movement allowed people to be optimistic. Referring to those who formerly sought relief in homeopathy as a last resort, Woodbury said the "invisible increment" now cast their lot with metaphysical healing. Woodbury attributed the loss of homeopathic patients not only to the "growing credulity" of the followers of new alternatives, but also to the increasing nihilism within the medical profession in general.[79] A significant number of physicians believed that with the exception of advances in surgery and a few notable successes such as salvarsan, vaccines, serum therapy, and insulin, there had been little advancement in therapeutics.[80] Whereas in the nineteenth century, homeopaths had presented themselves as a separate school of medicine, by the 1920s, distinctions between homeopaths and regulars were largely conflated in minds of the public. Not only did regulars and homeopaths borrow from each others' armamentaria, but homeopaths and mainstream physicians also belonged to the same professional organizations. Adding to the confusion, homeopaths often did not identify themselves as such to patients even when prescribing according to traditional homeopathic teachings. In the nineteenth century, people's dissatisfaction with the therapeutics of regular doctors worked to the advantage of homeopaths. Early-twentieth-century therapeutic nihilism worked against them. They were now part of the problem. One Philadelphia homeopath noted: "therapeutic nihilism is damning the medical profession and driving its clientele into the ranks of the drugless cults," a result, he said, of medical schools' subordination of therapeutics in their attempt to make "scientific physicians."[81] Compounding these problems, homeopaths with large and prosperous practices were the gatekeepers to wealthy patients, and often refused to provide Dennett with names.

Conrad Wesselhoeft, a Harvard graduate and influential Boston homeopath, called the Foundation's literature "very poor stuff" and hated its "cheap appeals to lay interest."[82] Both male and female practitioners mentioned the embarrassing decline in substance and form of homeopathic periodic literature.[83] And Wesselhoeft was "perfectly disgusted" with his colleagues in the IHA and AIH, finding their "politics, medical flag-waving . . . [and] the promotion of creeds instead of therapeutics," embarrassing.[84] Henry Houghton, who had one of the wealthiest homeopathic practices in Boston, declined to meet with Dennett.[85] Both Wesselhoeft and Houghton were members of the Massachusetts Medical Society, and according to Dr. Elizabeth Wright (later Hubbard), a friend of both men, the two "would hold back from anything that might prejudice regular medicine and the general public against them."[86] Neither Wesselhoeft nor Houghton wished to risk his good reputation by supporting an organization of extremists. They would wait and see.

Dr. Elizabeth Wright, however, was enthusiastic about the Foundation from her first meeting with Dennett. Recently arrived in Boston, with no established professional relationships, Wright was less cautious. Part of a new and severely diminished generation of women homeopaths, Wright was a graduate of Barnard College, and received her medical degree from the College of Physicians and Surgeons at Columbia University in 1921, the first class to matriculate women. After a two-year rotating internship at Bellevue Hospital, Wright joined the staff of Woodside Sanitarium for Nervous and Mental Diseases near Boston, which was headed by Swedenborgian homeopath Dr. Frank Wallace Patch. With Patch's encouragement, Wright traveled to Geneva and studied pure homeopathy under Dr. Pierre Schmidt and Dr. Emil Schlegel of Tubingen. Returning to Boston, Wright took charge of the homeopathic clinic at Massachusetts Memorial Hospital, and within a few years, attended the AFH post-graduate school. Although encouraged by her father to attend "the best of traditional medical schools," Wright was "born into homeopathy."[87] Homeopath Byron G. Clark not only assisted at her birth, but also cured Wright of various childhood illnesses, including tubercular cervical adenitis, malaria, and measles. According to Wright, during her internship at Bellevue, New York homeopath Rudolf Rabe cured her of a "violent delirious scarlet fever" with a single, high-potency dose of ammonium carbonicum.[88]

Wright's interest in homeopathy increased when she compared her positive responses to homeopathic treatment with the "paucity of therapeutic information" at Columbia Medical School. During her years as a medical student, Wright was frustrated by the lack of emphasis on therapeutics, which drove many students previously interested in general medicine into surgery or other specialties because there "was something definite to do for the patients." Wright said, "being a woman, and therefore a practical soul," she "hankered after the means of cure." Yet, according to Wright, therapeutic teaching consisted mostly of "hygiene, nursing procedures, diet, hydrotheraphy, etc." She was troubled by the lifelong sufferers of chronic indigestion or migraines who had been passed around from doctor to doctor with nothing but temporary relief of their symptoms. And she was particularly distressed when patients were told there was nothing wrong with them, based on the results of diagnostic procedures and laboratory tests, although they had abundant subjective symptoms and insisted they were truly sick.[89] In addition to her belief that homeopathic therapeutics would benefit such patients, Wright's professional opportunities as a homeopathic physician were plentiful. Her advocacy of homeopathy was not detrimental to her medical career.

After graduation and study in Europe, Wright was invited by Boston homeopath Alice H. Bassett to join her practice. According to Bassett, patients' demand for homeopathic physicians in Boston exceeded the supply of physicians. Wesselhoeft and Houghton were "submerged in work," and Bassett had appointments every fifteen minutes.[90] Wright was soon placed in charge of the homeopathic clinic at Massachusetts Memorial Hospital, and welcomed into the community of elite Boston homeopaths. During this time, she edited the *Homoeopathic Recorder*, the primary journal of Hahnemannians, and was an active member of the AIH, IHA, and AFH. Within a year of moving to Boston, Wright established a separate medical practice and was appointed to be one of four attending physicians at New England Hospital for Women and Children. Of the many physicians she interviewed, Mary Ware Dennett was especially impressed by Elizabeth Wright, describing her "extraordinarily fine mind," "youth," and "devotion to the highest type of homoeopathy." According to Dennett, Wright's office was "well equipped with all the required paraphernalia for complete physical examination," including a laboratory for "examinations of urine, blood, etc." Dennett hoped Wright's enthusiasm would be a "good antidote" to the discouragement of some of Boston's older homeopaths.[91]

Prognosis for Homeopathy

Pessimism over homeopathy's institutional future, and antagonism toward homeopathic institutions, organizations, or groups of physicians were common themes in most of the cities Dennett visited. In Chicago, the profession was hopelessly factionalized, a legacy from the days when as many as four homeopathic colleges competed for students, faculty, and funds. Both male and female homeopaths shared the sentiment of Dr. Charlotte Wandell who no longer had "faith in the ability of organizations to accomplish goals."[92] According to homeopath Mary E. Hanks, homeopaths in the city had not been "good business people—haven't known how to raise or to spend money."[93] But despite pessimism over the institutional decline of homeopathy, women's professional careers appeared to be thriving (like Wright's and Bassett's in Boston). In addition to her "large practice," Cleveland homeopath Alice Butler was president of the Board of Trustees of Women's Hospital, where one-third of the staff of the two-hundred-bed hospital were homeopaths. Homeopathic practitioner Mabelle Gilbert was chief of the hospital staff. Butler and Gilbert were active members of the Women's Hospital Association and often presented lectures at meetings attended by both homeopathic and regular physicians.[94] According to Dennett, both women "warmed" to the idea of the Foundation.

In Chicago, Dennett met jointly with homeopaths Julia C. Strawn, Lillian Thompson, and Frances Gage Hulbert. All had busy medical practices, and were actively involved in various local professional and civic organizations, including the Chicago Homoeopathic Society. Hulbert was president of the Women's After Dinner Club, a local society of physicians, nurses, and laypeople interested in homeopathy. Thompson headed two Chicago clinics—one on the South Side and another in conjunction with the Salvation Army. She was eagerly awaiting the arrival of a young woman intern from Cleveland to assist in her practice. The women readily provided Dennett with the names of patients they believed would be interested in the Foundation. According to her colleagues, Strawn had the most lucrative practice of Chicago's women physicians.[95]

In most of her interviews with women physicians in various locations, Dennett reported frequent interruptions, the need to wait for physicians to finish with patients, or meetings cut short due to previously scheduled appointments. Her assistant busy with patients, Mary E. Hanks allotted Dennett a half hour during which she "looked at her wrist watch and scanned her mail," behavior indicating both pressure for time as well as reluctance to be solicited for funds to support yet another potentially mismanaged homeopathic organization.[96]

During approximately two years' of fieldwork, Dennett interviewed homeopathic patients (thirty-two women and sixty-eight men) in Massachusetts, New York, New Jersey, Maryland, Pennsylvania, Ohio, and Illinois. Dennett variously described them as "comfortable," "well-to-do," or "wealthy." Most were middle age or older; and the men were lawyers, state senators, businessmen, investment bankers, pharmacists, chemists, and librarians. While one woman was a librarian and another a chemist, most were full-time homemakers involved in a variety of civic and volunteer organizations; a few were mothers of young children. Some were related to homeopathic practitioners or traveled in the same social circles as physicians.[97] They represented the Foundation's best hopes for success.

Analysis of Dennett's interviews reveals the various meanings of home-opathy to patients. In many cases, dedication to homeopathy itself was inci-dental to the loyalty patients felt toward individual physicians. Patients under the care of homeopaths nearing retirement felt some urgency to ensure that the same kind of care would be available from new physicians and were com-pletely responsive to Dennett's appeals on behalf of the Foundation. For example, Julia Loos's patients seemed particularly devoted to her and at a loss when she moved her practice from Harrisburg, Pennsylvania. Mrs. C. M. Sigler said her husband was a "tremendous enthusiast about Dr. Loos," and that she herself, "misses Dr. Loos sadly and does not know to whom else to turn." Mrs. B. F. Snavely of Lancaster, Pennsylvania, also keenly felt her loss and "still depends upon her for prescribing by mail when necessary. Both women responded positively to the Foundation's programs when Dennett reminded them one of its aims is "to make more Dr. Looses." New York invest-ment banker Louis Musil whose family members were patients of homeopath Stuart Close did not know where he should turn "if Dr. Close were to die." Musil said Close knew all about his family "and their entire physical makeup and predispositions."[98]

While such patients were sympathetic toward the Foundation because they valued individual physicians either as close personal friends or because they "liked the way they doctored," an equal number of men and women sup-ported the Foundation's plan to educate "good" homeopathic doctors on ideo-logical grounds. Mrs. Frank A. Hall of Montclair, New Jersey, informed Dennett she was only interested in "genuine Hahnemannian Homoeopathy . . . It will be a waste of time to discuss any other form." Mrs. William S. Hal-lowell of Philadelphia claimed she was "deeply interested in homeopathy, that is in real homeopathy." Hallowell questioned Dennett on the kind of teachers in the Foundation's school, asking: "Are they just modernists who have merely lessened allopathic dosing . . . or true homeopaths." Retired Navy offi-cer, Captain Harrison A. Bispham, a patient of Fredericka Gladwin's in Philadelphia, said he "appreciates homeopathy and knows the difference between the real sort and nominal sort." Mrs. John S. Reed of Waltham, Massachusetts, called herself a "true-blue homoeopath," one who knows the difference between "a mongrel and a real one."[99] But Mrs. Leopold Auer's comment amused Dennett most and perhaps reflects the feelings of many homeopathic patients at that time. Married to a noted violinist, Mrs. Auer was of Russian ancestry and had been raised in Europe where she "heard much" about homeopathy. She used her own "little kit of remedies," and talked about homeopathy to her friends. But according to Dennett, Mrs. Auer had "no real understanding of the subject." Attempting to reproduce her accent in writing, Dennett quoted Auer's answer to the question of whether she believed in homeopathy: "Homoeopahtee? Yes I believe in it, also Allopahtee sometimes. But I do not *first* believe in Homoeopahtee, I take the remedies. They do me good. *Then* I believe." Auer read with interest the booklet Dennett gave her, *Homoeopathy: A Pamphlet for the People*, asking Dennett to send her fifty more copies to give to her friends.[100]

Like Auer, most patients Dennett interviewed based their support of homeopathy on personal experience. In Illinois, Dennett met with Mr. and Mrs. Walter A. Sheriffs and Mrs. R. J. Gaudy. According to Dennett, there was "no great wealth in either family." They were "the sort who have one housemaid," but they were young, intelligent parents of small children, and "ideal people to reach, so far as spreading the news of the Foundation is concerned." Mrs. Sheriffs credited homeopath Harvey Farrington for ending her long battle with "the exzema (sic)-asthma combination," a condition she believed was inherited. Worried her "little daughter" had similar tendencies, Mrs. Sheriffs was particularly interested in the potential of homeopathy to "gradually uproot" inherited chronic diseases from families. Mrs. Gaudy had been a patient of Dr. Farrington's for only two years. But having suffered from sinus trouble and the "probings, sprayings," and "all manner of miseries under old school treatment," Gaudy had been "straightened out" by Dr. Farrington. And although she knew little of the principles of homeopathy, she was "keen to learn."[101]

John S. Dove Jr., a member of the advisory board of Philadelphia's Women's Southern Hospital, was enthusiastic about the Foundation's plan to educate laypeople. Dove converted to homeopathy after his "baby's life was saved years ago"; and, after having been "given up for dead," Dove himself had been cured of cirrhosis of the liver by homeopath Raymond Harris. Dove asked Dennett for Foundation literature to distribute to hospital associates. Bruce Walter of Pittsburgh, Pennsylvania, suffered with "chronic headaches" as a young man. Raised in an "allopathic family," Walter took "all sorts of dope," yet his headaches persisted. He became interested in homeopathy after meeting a homeopathic physician socially. Thereafter, he became the patient of Dr. Crowley, whose "wonderfuly (sic) fine" prescribing cured him. Walter told Dennett his employer, Lawrence E. Riddle may "give handsomely" to the Foundation. Riddle's daughter was being treated by Dr. Cowley for Bright's disease. According to Walter, she was making "real progress," after being told by "old school" physicians she could not last two years. "If she is really cured her father is likely to have a tremendous appreciation of homoeopathy."[102]

The cure of children under homeopathic care, when all previous therapies had failed, often led to their lifelong advocacy of homeopathy and the conversion of parents. Mrs. J. Waddell had been a homeopathic patient from the age of twelve. Nearing age seventy, Waddell and her husband, a civil engineer and "a very active businessman," traveled widely and had many acquaintances. Dennett hoped Waddell would spread news of the Foundation. Dennett found Waddell a "friendly critic," who said homeopathic physicians should take time to explain their treatment of babies to mothers—"an intelligent mother is the doctor's best ally." Waddell believed by increasing mothers' understanding of homeopathy, the promotion of homeopathy among laypeople "would increase perceptibly."[103] Other patients were sharply critical of homeopathic doctors, arguing physicians did not explain homeopathic therapeutics to patients, ignored physical exams, and paid little attention to preventive medicine.

Alma Hiller, a chemist at Rockefeller Institute in New York City, was most interested in the Foundation's plan for research, which would elevate homeopathy to the level of a "demonstrable science." Hiller told Dennett she knew several "good" homeopaths, and with the exception of her personal physician, they prescribed "in silence," leaving the patient "in the dark as to what it is all about." The family of wealthy, retired businessman Decatur Sawyer had been under the care of several well-known homeopaths. Sawyer approved of the Foundation's plan to educate more "thorough-going homeopaths," telling Dennett he had observed the "superficial attention which many supposedly good homoeopaths give to their patients." Dennett sympathized with Sawyer's criticism. Having been under the care of some of the "finest homoeopathic physicians in the land," Dennett never received a complete physical examination. According to Dennett, she underwent several unnecessary surgeries resulting from physicians' neglect of proper examinations and treatment. In her opinion, physicians who based treatment solely on symptoms missed important opportunities to "create and conserve" health.[104]

According to Walter Sheriffs, Illinois homeopath Harvey Farrington paid no attention to diet. Sheriffs believed it lessened Farrington's "all-round . . . usefulness to the patient." In Philadelphia, Dennett met with Edward C. Bostock, "the very picture of the rich young businessman, alone in his fine big office." Bostock, who had "always been a homoeopath," told Dennett all the physicians he knew were "considerably unsatisfactory." He believed many of the "best homoeopaths" had been "too indifferent to hygiene, and other means for creating and conserving health." Hermann L. Grote of Pittsburgh, Pennsylvania, believed the Foundation's plan to educate the laity would help patients protect themselves from poor therapeutic practices. Grote criticized the "theoretical" rather than "practical" prescribing of local homeopath Dr. Cowley. Grote cited one instance when a patient of Cowley's grew worse rather than better after Cowley prescribed the "best indicated similar remedy." Cowley let the patient "get next door to death, still insisting that he was improving because he had been given the right remedy."[105] Despite such criticisms, and perhaps because of them, patients Dennett interviewed were overwhelmingly supportive of the Foundation's program to ensure a proper education in homeopathy for a new generation of homeopathic physicians.

Patients generally appreciated the Foundation's nonpartisan approach to unify a fractious profession in order to preserve homeopathy. Harry Parkhurst, brother of Baltimore homeopath Alice Parkhurst, complained homeopaths in his city had been "lazy and quarrelsome for years . . . Forty years ago they had all the best people in Baltimore behind them. Now they are losing out fast." In his opinion, only "vigorous demand" by laypeople would induce doctors to "give good service."[106] But the "vigorous demand" Mary Ware Dennett and Julia Green anticipated from specific groups of patients never materialized. She found Swedenborgian patients particularly "hard-boiled and indifferent."[107]

Followers of Emanuel Swedenborg had been enthusiastic disciples of Hahnemann in the nineteenth century. They were prominent homeopathic physicians, trustees of homeopathic colleges, homeopathic pharmacists, and dedicated patients. But the outcome of Dennett's visit to Swedenborgian communities in Bryn Athyn, Pennsylvania, revealed a lack of interest in homeopathy among both the younger and older generations. A meeting in Glenview, Illinois, in February 1927 elicited a more positive response—about thirty-five attendees asked "many interesting questions" and wanted additional literature on the Foundation." In Cambridge, Massachusetts, Dennett met with Mrs. John C. Moses, patient of Swedenborgian homeopath Dr. Florence Taft. Moses told Dennett she personally knew between one hundred and one hundred-fifty lay homeopaths through her "New Church connections." As president of the Women's New Church Alliance, Mrs. Moses offered to send invitations to all her homeopathic friends for a future meeting. But expectations far exceeded the twenty-five people who attended the gathering at the home of Rev. William L. Worcester in April 1927. Mrs. Moses speculated that the reason for the low attendance was because there were "so few *real* homoeopaths in Cambridge [author's italics]."[108] Dennett's and Green's expectations of large donations from homeopathy's wealthier patients were also unfulfilled.

In the Boston suburb of Brookline, Dennett interviewed Mrs. George D. Pike whose "beautiful home" rested atop "one of the Brookline hills." Dennett characterized Pike as "completely the leisure sort of woman. I found her placidly playing Mah Jong when I arrived." A patient of Dr. Turner, Pike was twice cured of pneumonia, and was "interested" and "appreciative" of homeopathy. But after apologizing to Dennett that her chauffeur was off for the day and could not drive her back to the city, Pike told Dennett she "absolutely couldn't" contribute financially to the Foundation. Disappointed, Dennett speculated that perhaps Pike had "no income of her own, and . . . a tightwad allopathic husband! You never can tell." Chicago homeopath Julia Strawn provided Dennett with a letter of introduction to her wealthiest patient—William Wrigley of chewing gum fame.[109] But despite Strawn's recommendation, Wrigley refused to see Dennett. Remembering Wrigley's generous donation to the Voluntary Parenthood League, Dennett believed Wrigley "steers away from the experimental stages of any work." However, Julia Green learned Wrigley was "disgusted" with homeopathic politics and the bitter relations between homeopaths in Chicago, and he lacked faith in the ability of homeopaths to work together for a common purpose.[110] According to Mr. Ehrhart of Ehrhart and Karl Homeopathic Pharmacy in Chicago, Wrigley withdrew from several previously proposed homeopathic "projects," not only because of factionalism, but also because "they were not teaching true Homoeopathy." And Chicago homeopath A. H. Gordon proffered yet another theory for Wrigley's refusal to meet with Dennett. Noting Wrigley's $200,000 gift to Chicago Memorial Hospital arranged by Julia Strawn, Gordon said Wrigley had a "strong instinct toward self-advertising" and wanted his money to attract the spotlight to himself. Whatever Wrigley's true feelings about homeopathy, philanthropists usually supported projects whose chances for success were high, judiciously putting their funds behind mainstream developments in professionalism such as hospitals, university medical centers, and nursing education where "short-term change might be achieved."[111]

Although Raymond Pitcairn's father had liberally supported James Tyler Kent's Post-Graduate School of Homeopathics in Philadelphia in the 1890s, his son—the young, wealthy leader of the Bryn Athyn, Pennsylvania, Swedenborgian community—refused to meet with Dennett despite two special delivery letters sent to his office and home. According to Dr. Louis Olds who knew Pitcairn, the latter had "slight" interest in homeopathy and was "completely absorbed in Church and his own affairs."[112] Dennett and Green's hopes for a large endowment from John D. Rockefeller—homeopathy's most famous patient—rested on the latter's close friendship with homeopathic physician Hamilton Biggar. But Rockefeller's personal secretary W. H. Richardson was not encouraging, noting Dr. Biggar had tried "several times" without success to "get him [Rockefeller] to do something for homeopathy," and that Rockefeller's son would "probably have none of it."[113] Julia Green planned to write to Biggar, enlisting his help, but when Biggar died in November 1926, she believed the Foundation's best hopes for Rockefeller money died with him.

Dennett wrote to Green: "It is maddening to think of all that vast wealth sitting there back of that dried-up old man, when it ought to be let out into channels that lead to the salvation and enrichment of life on a big scale."[114]

In spite of Biggar's friendship with Rockefeller and of the latter's personal dedication to homeopathy, it is highly unlikely the doctor could have influenced his friend regarding the Foundation. Beginning in the last decade of the nineteenth century, Frederick T. Gates, Rockefeller's chief financial adviser and architect of his philanthropies, directed Rockefeller funds. Carefully negotiating between his employer's allegiance to homeopathy and his own idea of medical progress, Gates effectively mobilized the power of Rockefeller's wealth behind scientific, technological medicine, providing a leadership followed by other foundations and wealthy individuals.[115]

A Ladies-Only Affair

By the spring of 1926, subscriptions to AFH publications numbered 237.[116] Although Dennett's powers of persuasion converted many a reluctant physician to support the Foundation's cause, income barely covered basic operating expenses and Dennett's salary. The board expressed appreciation for Dennett's work, but doubted the wisdom of keeping her on the payroll given the Foundation's precarious financial status. Green and Loos defended Dennett's value to the organization, knowing trustees had paid little attention to Dennett's lengthy and detailed reports and her role in helping Green formulate fundraising plans. While trustees acknowledged that the finance committee had been "a dead failure," they blamed Dennett for the lack of contributions.[117]

As Regina Morantz-Sanchez and other scholars have noted, by the second decade of the twentieth century, "scientific medicine" had become a predominantly masculine profession. A cultural reaction against the "new woman" between 1910 and 1930, emphasizing women's central role as wife and mother, made women's prominence in "masculinized" professions or organizations appear deviant, lowering the status of such organizations.[118] In January 1926, Green confided to Dennett that "some of the men" had become critical of women's prominence as trustees and teachers in the post-graduate school. Having experienced similar negative reactions to women trustees and Foundation teachers among male physicians in particular locations, Dennett responded that such feeling was "old-fashioned" yet "inevitable."[119] But some women homeopaths were also convinced the lack of important male physicians on the board and teaching staff of the Foundation lowered its "standing" and "contributed to the general feebleness" of homeopathy's status. Admitting her opinion of the Foundation was probably influenced by the general conservatism in

Boston, Alice Bassett called it a "ladies-only affair."[120] At a time when women lost their leadership positions to men—Sanger's American Birth Control League being one example—the high profile of women in the Foundation became a detriment.[121] New board member Elizabeth Wright agreed with Bassett. Insisting a "man" should represent the Foundation, Wright said she heard much criticism of the AFH as a "woman's institution . . . it is a dangerous thing to be a woman's institution even if it is run by Amazons . . . It just adds another slur . . . We hate to have it so . . . but . . . if you want to sell something, you have to do something to sell it, and the people object to our being a woman's institution."[122] Besides the growing unrest regarding women's high profile roles in the organization, Wright and others criticized the Foundation's promotion of lay leagues.

AFH founders had envisioned equal roles for physicians and laypeople in the promotion of homeopathy at a time when complex, specialized medical knowledge, lay deference, and institutionalized forms of dependence increasingly formed the basis of physicians' status and authority. The conscious creation of an elite occupational class widened the distance between patients and doctors. Eager to conform to mainstream professional norms, some homeopaths were reluctant to support an organization they considered detrimental to their individual interests and to what remained of the homeopathic profession.[123]

Trustee Royal S. Hayes thought laymen's work complicated relations with the majority of homeopaths and regular physicians, believing patient education was best conducted by individual physicians among their patients. Wright said doctors in New England resented being approached by a laywoman, saying she heard much criticism of Dennett. "I think if you told certain people . . . that Mrs. Dennett will be finished by September 1, they would be delighted." Although she had originally favored the Foundation's plan to educate patients, Wright had changed her mind. She now considered the promotion of lay leagues a "bad mistake . . . Why if people in regular medicine begin proselytizing among the laymen and pandering among the laymen . . . they immediately get tagged as almost patent medicine; I mean, it isn't scientific, it isn't done."[124]

Although Green and Loos defended lay education in general and Dennett's value to the organization in particular, the board voted to terminate Dennett's contract, considering Dennett's work a practical failure and her position as representative a hindrance to future progress.[125] Dennett resigned as special representative of the AFH on July 2, 1927. Determined to further the Foundation's cause by any means possible, Green relinquished her position as chair. She urged the board to replace her with a man, and in January

1927, Dr. Herbert A. Roberts, secretary of the IHA and one of the original trustees of the AFH, was elected to the position.[126]

By the end of the decade, the makeup of the board had changed. Julia Green's "self-sacrificing" style of leadership conflicted with the ideas of Elizabeth Wright who became an influential and popular trustee. Wright believed in committees and a bureaucratic style of organization.[127] Although she did not say it outright, Elizabeth Wright assumed the organization's slow growth was largely due to the "inefficient," "feminine," and distinctly "old-fashioned" leadership style of Julia Green. Green was the only original trustee remaining on a board strongly opposed to the promotion of lay education through the development of lay leagues. At Green's urging, the trustees agreed to let the issue "simmer," neither promoting nor abandoning the commitment to lay education. However, by de-emphasizing lay work and electing males as prominent representatives, the Foundation survived, however marginally, as an organization.

The ongoing debates between Julia Green and Elizabeth Wright on issues of organization and focus were not based simply on differences in personality or style. They represented changing concepts of feminism in early-twentieth-century American culture. Julia Green was part of a previous generation of women physicians who felt more connected to the female community at large. Nineteenth-century social feminists like Green often felt forced to choose between marriage and children or a career, believing the two incompatible. They derived fulfillment from their contributions to the welfare of the community, the sisterhood of women, and to their professions. Their careers were a primary source of both intellectual and emotional fulfillment.[128]

In 1930, Elizabeth Wright married Benjamin A. Hubbard. She was part of a new generation of women professionals who were less likely to view family and public life as mutually exclusive. Moving to New York City where her husband was on the faculty of Columbia University, Wright Hubbard became the mother of five children while continuing to practice medicine and actively participate in homeopathic organizations.[129] She would not have defined herself as a feminist; women of her generation came of age in a cultural climate that downplayed female relationships and rejected public feminism. Sometimes arrogant, they were often unwilling to acknowledge the struggles of older women or believe in the necessity for continued promotion of female goals.[130] Not only had she successfully combined a satisfying and full personal life with a career but also in her experience, she suffered no barriers to educational and professional opportunities. Educated at one of the country's best medical schools, well received by an overwhelmingly male student body, and respected by colleagues in her profession, she believed women who worked hard enough and were serious about a medical career would not be hindered by lack of opportunity. To use more recent terminology, Wright Hubbard did not view the personal as political. Having made it in a man's world, she believed individual perseverance and ability were the keys to accomplishing one's goals. Like many professionals of Wright Hubbard's generation, her reference group was male. She enjoyed the admiration of male colleagues, and clearly preferred working with men, finding their methods more direct and efficient.

Although Hayes believed the Washington Layman's League would die a "natural death," it was among eleven lay leagues still in existence in 1961. Women continued to be elected to the board, although none served as chair for the next several decades. Julia Green remained active in the Foundation throughout her life—teaching in the post-graduate school from 1931 to 1951 and developing a curriculum for the first layman's course instituted in 1945. She persistently promoted lay leagues, believing the survival of homeopathy depended upon an educated laity who would demand and support "true" homeopaths. Corresponding with a colleague in 1957, Green reflected on the outcome of the AFH election in 1927.

> This left me with a deep feeling of responsibility, a feeling I have carried with me ever since.—I was on the Board with no one else to make the effort to keep the policies of the Foundation either understood or carried out. I think I should have resigned then and there if something inside of me did not commend me to keep on. In fact this feeling has remained with me throughout the Foundation's existence and will not let go.[131]

While it is logical to assume medical practices of women homeopaths in the 1930s and thereafter suffered from declining authority and interest in homeopathic medicine, just the opposite is true—their dual identity as physicians and homeopaths was an advantage. Lacking understanding of the meaning of homeopathy, patients simply wanted "good" physicians, those who cared and cured. Avid Hahnemannian patients continued to support "good" homeopaths—those adhering to traditional homeopathic philosophy and therapeutics. And patients who were ambivalent about homeopathy continued to patronize physicians with whom they had enjoyed long-standing and rewarding relationships.

Although institutional opportunities for women disappeared with the demise of homeopathic medical schools and hospitals, their situation was not appreciably worse, and was perhaps better in some respects, than that of women regular physicians. Although the precariousness of the AFH made it more vulnerable to charges that its status would be compromised by women's prominence and lay work, women continued to present papers at meetings of national and local homeopathic medical societies, serve on committees and executive boards, and edit and publish in major homeopathic journals.[132] Women in mainstream medicine, however, were often outspoken in their conviction that they were denied equal status in a profession dominated by men, claiming "Men do not want women in their institutions and organizations except as subordinates and auxiliaries."[133] In contrast, homeopaths in the IHA elected Grace Stevens of Massachusetts the first woman president of a national homeopathic organization in 1930, and Sarah M. Hobson edited the *Journal of the American Institute of Homoeopathy*. In 1945 Elizabeth Wright Hubbard was elected president of the IHA, and in 1959 she became president of the larger American Institute of Homoeopathy. Women's choice of homeopathy in the twentieth century was not necessarily a conscious strategy to increase professional opportunities. But by straddling the margins of American medicine, women enhanced their potential to build lucrative medical practices, while taking advantage of leadership opportunities increasingly unavailable to women who remained firmly within the bounds of orthodoxy.

Epilogue	Twentieth-Century Transformation and Rebirth

HISTORIANS OF WOMEN in medicine have assumed that by the 1890s, when the implications and meanings of scientific medicine elevated the authority of regular medicine, women regulars were "the only individuals who commanded much respect from the orthodox professionals."[1] This view is challenged, however, by the decline in homeopathic distinctiveness in education and therapeutic practices. In the opinion of William Osler, "the differences which, in matters of treatment, separate members of the rational school are not greater than those which separate some of us from our homeopathic brethren."[2] The turn of the century practice of Eliza Taylor Ransom is but one example of the dissolving boundaries between homeopathy and orthodoxy and its significance for the careers of women homeopathic practitioners.

Although Ransom graduated in 1900 from the homeopathic medical school at Boston University and taught histology there for several years, she also studied neurology with William Osler at Johns Hopkins in 1902.[3] She became a prominent leader in homeopathic organizations, professional women's clubs, civic organizations, and the twilight sleep and suffrage movements. Ransom investigated twilight sleep methods in collaboration with John Osborn Polack, a leading regular obstetrician and educator in New York.[4] At the turn of the century, Ransom and her female homeopathic colleagues in Boston outnumbered women regular physicians. They constituted 35 percent of the homeopathic profession in the city, and were notable for their lucrative medical practices.[5] A 1904 news article on the earnings of professional women in Boston noted that along with Ransom, homeopath Eliza B. Cahill had "one of the finest practices in the city," netting $12,000 per year. Homeopath Sarah Windsor had a "fine class of patients who pay high fees," netting the practitioner $6,000 to $7,000.[6] Rather than suffering from lack of respect or from marginalization by their association with homeopathy, Ransom and many other women homeopaths enjoyed the patronage of wealthy patients, cordial professional relations with regulars, and continued a tradition of leadership in homeopathic organizations. They joined alumnae associations and women's medical societies previously closed to them. During World War I, homeopaths Cornelia C. Brant, Adelaide Brown, and Florence N. Ward served on the Committee of Women Physicians of the General Medical Board of the Council of National Defense with Rosalie Slaughter Morton and other notable women regulars.[7] As Naomi Rogers has pointed out, homeopaths were prominent during this period in American public life. For example, Warren G. Harding brought his family's homeopathic physician to the White House during his term as president, and when Calvin Coolidge assumed the presidency, war hero and homeopathic physician Joel Boone was a close adviser.[8]

While the late-nineteenth-century scientific revolution changed the structure and financing of medical institutions and contributed to the decline of homeopathic institutions, it had less effect on patients' choice of physicians. Patients continued to patronize homeopaths with whom they had long-standing relationships and whose therapies they thought "worked," recommending such doctors to friends. And while by the early 1900s, laboratory advances produced impressive accomplishments, such as diphtheria antitoxin, various serums, and vaccines, there was little immediate effect on physicians' everyday practices with patients.

As historian Harry Marks demonstrates, proprietary compounds manufactured by drug firms were 72 percent of the U.S. drug market in 1900. They were effectively promoted along with nostrums claiming cures for all manners of ills. Physicians as well as laypeople were the targets of advertising campaigns by manufacturers whose claims for drug efficacy were untested and unproven, since the ingredients of these products were known only to manufacturers.[9] Both homeopaths and regulars decried the escalating commercialism in medicine. Homeopath Eugene Underhill Jr., complained:

> People who have never even matriculated at a medical college will come in and recite their piece, telling us the most up to date and accredited manner of treating our patients . . . physicians . . . are preyed upon, even coerced by large manufacturing interests, not for welfare of humanity and the protection of the public . . . but in their own interest and solely for the cold coin of the realm.[10]

Therapeutic reformers sought to control the introduction and promotion of new drugs, as well as foster a critical attitude among practitioners to ensure their effective and appropriate use. While there were a few successful clinical studies performed under the auspices of the AMA's Council on Pharmacy and Chemistry (1905), therapeutic reformers of the 1920s still lamented their lack of progress. The majority of physicians continued to choose drugs based on personal and limited clinical experience as well as testimonials from others.[11] In this environment, it is no wonder that homeopaths' knowledge of remedy composition and a materia medica based on a tradition of drug testing remained a source of pride to many.

For many decades the work of laboratory scientists and hospital clinicians held little relevance to the everyday treatment of patients. Although new scientific products were lauded as examples of medical progress, their practical benefit was often limited. For example, although Rockefeller Institute introduced the first successful serum to treat pneumonia in 1913, potentially harmful allergic reactions and the required intravenous administration necessitated patient supervision in hospitals. Subsequent discoveries of various types of pneumonia required treatment by type-specific serum. Yet, few laboratories were equipped for pneumococcal typing. Fifteen years after its introduction, the high cost and special requirements for administering the serum deterred its use among all but a handful of practitioners with access to laboratories and hospital facilities.[12] Scholars have noted, that early-twentieth-century "aspirations of science so far exceeded its visible accomplishments that any confidence in the authority of science seems misplaced."[13]

For the majority of physicians, homeopathic and regular, the laboratory was an abstract emblem of scientific progress, but a concrete means of confirming diagnoses and determining the efficacy of treatment. For example, in November 1927, San Francisco homeopath Laura B. Hurd took over the case of a sixty-two-year-old man who complained of severe pain four months after his previous physician had performed an operation to drain an abscess in his chest. Although Hurd treated the patient with homeopathic remedies according to the principle of symptom similarity, she turned to laboratory analyses to aid her diagnosis and help her determine if the remedies she prescribed changed the patient's condition. At the conclusion of treatment, Hurd compared X-rays ordered by her patient's former physician with films she ordered in January, confirming "an infectious process" but showing improvement in both the pleura and lung tissue. Bacteriological examination of sputum, taken at intervals, revealed no tubercle bacilli. The blood Wasserman was negative, and Hurd compared erythrocytes and leukocytes in the blood to previous blood assays. Urinary analysis showed evidence of a little albumen, amorphous phosphates, and a few triple phosphate crystals. Based on the combination of calcified pleura, pleural thickening, and scarring in the lung roots, bronchial and lung tissue, Hurd concluded her patient suffered from a lung infection.[14] Throughout the course of treatment, Hurd changed or selected remedies based on the patient's observable symptoms according to homeopathic principles. For Hurd and many homeopaths, discoveries emanating from laboratories, especially research in immunology, confirmed the efficacy of minute doses and the continued relevance of the homeopathic pharmacopoeia of drugs.

Although the closing of homeopathic medical schools effectively ended homeopathy as a route to a regular medical career for women, women did not necessarily abandon their affiliation with homeopathy. According to the AIH directory of 1941, women homeopaths in the United States numbered 471, compared to 865 in 1925. Their continued association with homeopathy and the patronage of patients as late as the 1940s highlights the importance of personal experience, family influence and tradition, and the primacy of the doctor/patient relationship in the day-to-day practice of medicine. Although "American Medicine" in the twentieth century was a growing scientific, political, economic, and social force, medicine (writ small) was and is intensely personal. Given the general lack of drug knowledge and established guidelines for appropriate clinical application, decisions of what "worked"—for homeopaths as well as regulars—were based on the experiences of individual patients and physicians. Although older homeopathic institutions gradually disappeared, new ones developed, and the practice of homeopathy continued, however variously defined and restricted by the declining population of practitioners.

Rebirth

When a new generation of young people "discovered" homeopathy in the late 1960s and early 1970s, the AFH and affiliated lay leagues were primary sources of information, education, and support. During the years between 1930 and 1970, the AFH and league members (who were mostly women) encouraged the close association of patients and physicians. Sustaining and promoting a different understanding of disease etiology and therapeutics, they united advocates in a wide-ranging national and even international homeopathic community. For them, the triumph of orthodox medicine was not a scientific victory but a political one. Claiming that scientific discovery merely reinforced the power of unseen, nonmaterial life forces, they viewed the rising power and mutual interests of the American Medical Association and pharmaceutical industry as evidence that monetary profit rather than pure science determined medical orthodoxy.

Throughout these years, Hahnemannians were outspoken critics of local health authorities and medical practices. Leagues and the homeopathic community in general constituted a separate society, one in which members could discuss their ideas about medicine, health, and the failures of American democracy without being called crackpots. Their publications informed readers of "ineffective drugs," "false and misleading" advertising by drug companies, iatrogenic disease caused by physicians' improper use of drugs, as well as detrimental side effects of new "wonder drugs" such as penicillin and the sulfonamides.[15] Articles warned of the dangers of biomedical technology such as the X ray, criticized the fragmentation of medical care spurred by specialization, and reported on the corrupting influence of commercial interests on doctors. Most Hahnemannians opposed the compulsory vaccination of children against communicable diseases such as tetanus, diphtheria, and polio, believing them not only harmful but also a prime example of commercialism in medicine. As one physician put it, drug companies convinced physicians, boards of health, and the public into believing they were interested in the "welfare of humanity and the protection of the public" whereas their primary interests were "solely for the cold coin of the realm."[16]

During the 1950s and 1960s, Hahnemannians were active in organizations opposing the fluoridation of public water supplies in various communities. Calling it "mass medication . . . sanctioned by Government," they viewed any compulsory programs, including vaccination, as "mad attempts " by modern medical research to "standardize man" and violate personal liberty, "the most fundamental of human rights."[17] As the environmental movement gained strength in the wake of Rachel Carson's *Silent Spring* (1962), Hahnemannian publications and league newsletters focused on potential health hazards of hormones and antibiotics added to animal feed, as well as harmful effects from supposedly beneficial insecticides, fertilizers, and food preservatives. During this time, the Hahnemannian message was clear. Individuals must be vigilant. They must educate themselves on matters of health, recognizing that government health agencies, physicians, scientific experts, and others charged with the public's welfare could not be trusted.

Although the particular health threats were new, the libertarian and anti-materialist language of an earlier generation of homeopathic advocates resonated with the counterculture youth of the sixties and seventies who were convinced of the moral bankruptcy of established institutions and authority. In her 1960 address as president of the American Institute of Homoeopathy, Elizabeth Wright Hubbard emphasized the constitutional rights of "We, the people, as patients: to preserve health and resist the comodification of health by 'big business.'" She invoked the values of human freedom, the protection of the individual, and the rights of minorities as the "precious heritage" of democracy in its "original Jeffersonian form."[18] With the growth of the civil rights and feminist movements during this period, language defending individual and minority rights acquired new meaning. Homeopathy's identity as persecuted minority—outsider to mainstream medicine—greatly enhanced its appeal.[19]

In February 1969, homeopathy received national attention when an article titled, "Homoeopathy—A Neglected Medical Art" appeared in *Prevention* magazine. Published by Rodale Press, *Prevention* was the bible of self-help health advocates and natural foods enthusiasts, many of whom were also members of homeopathic lay leagues. By the beginning of the 1970s, the American Foundation for Homoeopathy was flooded with requests for literature and locations of homeopathic physicians, in addition to information on how to obtain domestic medical kits. Membership in lay leagues rose dramatically, with "so many young people coming to . . . meetings" that leagues were "hard put to accommodate them."[20] Gradually, leagues gave way to homeopathic study groups. Whereas leagues had emphasized patient education in homeopathic principles and philosophy, study groups focused on self-treatment—participants considered themselves practitioners rather than "patients."

To a new generation of young people, homeopathy represented personal freedom, self-reliance, empowerment, and a less expensive alternative to mainstream medicine. For physicians and other health care professionals discouraged and disappointed by mainstream medicine, homeopathy provided a less technological, less hierarchical, and less authoritarian means of practice. And for second-wave feminists, homeopathy offered an alternative to authoritarian and elitist values of mainstream medicine. As predominately white, middle-class women developed a new style of politics to redress the imbalance of power in both their professional and personal lives, many rejected the values of the predominantly male medical establishment, considering it a unique vehicle of female oppression and domination.

As one strand of the feminist revolution of the 1960s, the women's health movement encompassed several goals, including the demystification of medical knowledge and demedicalization of natural life events such as childbirth and menopause. Feminists demanded safer and more effective methods of birth control, and sought to remove the control exercised by doctors over reproductive technology. They challenged the superiority of doctor's so-called objective clinical knowledge over subjective knowledge based on women's own experiences of their bodies. Women organized self-help groups in which they shared knowledge and validated each other's experiences.[21] The corresponding increase in homeopathic study groups comprised mostly of women in the 1970s and 1980s, was in large part fueled by the politics of feminism.[22]

During her 1980 internship at Saint Clare's Hospital in Schenectady, New York, Lisa Harvey acquired a reputation for spending time with people, listening to them—and, running behind schedule.[23] Harvey was interested in a type of patient care that paid attention to the nutritional, emotional, psychological, and social needs influencing patients' health. Becoming frustrated with the antibiotics that were "thrown" at people, Harvey said she questioned herself every day about whether she was adhering to the physicians' primary dictum to "first do no harm." In 1982, Harvey moved to Berkeley, California, epicenter of the radical student movement, joining the staff of the Berkeley Women's Health Collective. There she was able to "listen to women's concerns and pay attention to their words." The collective was nonhierarchical, feminist, and cooperative with all personnel receiving approximately the same salary. Harvey viewed herself not as an "expert" or "Boss" but as a teacher and guide to patients. She first heard about homeopathy from several patients who were members of a homeopathic study group in Oakland. At that time, Harvey had become interested in "energetic medicine," which she defined as "a therapy that supports the body's own healing energy through nonmaterial means . . . [working] . . . on an energetic rather than a physical level." Homeopathy's metaphysical principles interested her and she joined the Oakland study group. Although one member was a nurse and another a nurse practitioner, most were not health professionals. Together they studied cases and developed ideas about appropriate homeopathic remedies. Consistent with feminist values, the collaborative nature and lack of hierarchy in most study groups also characterized some homeopathic medical practices.

Lia Bello began her career early in the 1970s as a nurse at the Greater Southeast Community Hospital in Washington, D.C., and believed she could make a difference in healing by paying attention to patients' words and their emotional needs.[24] However, Bello found little time to listen to and talk with patients given her many hospital responsibilities. Idealistic and eager to collaborate with physicians on patient care, she grew frustrated at doctors' lack of interest in what nurses had to say or in the notes they carefully recorded on patients' charts. A self-described "hippy" and feminist, Bello first heard the word "homeopathy" from a clerk in a local health food store. Intrigued, Bello paid a visit to the nearby office of the National Center for Homoeopathy. After a program of independent study and attending a course in homeopathy for medical professionals at the NCH, Bello became an apprentice to Washington, D.C. homeopathic physician David Wember. She later joined

Wember's practice along with well-known lay prescriber Catherine Coulter, who had studied homeopathy in France. With an emphasis on the patient's emotional state and temperament in prescribing homeopathic remedies, their homeopathic practice corresponded to Bello's own ideas on the role of emotions in healing. Increasingly conscious of herself as a "spiritual being" during this period in her life, homeopathy offered Bello metaphysical understanding of illness and health. As part of a team where doctor, nurse, and lay prescriber contributed equally to discussions of patients' cases, homeopathic practice provided the egalitarianism and collaboration for which she had been searching.

Legacy

Today, homeopathy is one of the most popular alternative or complementary therapies to mainstream medicine in the United States. Clearly, homoeopathy's proponents and practitioners consider homoeopathy useful in preventing illness and managing disease. Throughout its history, however, it was also a tool for conceptualizing and criticizing not only American medicine but also society in general.

Prominent critics of twentieth-century American culture, including Christopher Lasch, Jackson Lears, and others, believe that growing fragmentation, commercialization, and secularization of modern life and its "complacent creed of progress," stimulated yearnings for the "authentic, the natural, and the real."[25] In the late twentieth century, these desires invigorated a plethora of unconventional approaches to healing, including naturopathy, acupuncture, and homoeopathy as well as "holistic" therapies such as a reflexology, massage, therapeutic touch, and herbalism, among others.[26] Common to all is the idea that the body possesses an innate wisdom that causes it to strive toward perfect health. According to this theory, an individual's internal drive, "energy," or vital life force, is aided by the "natural" therapies of holistic systems and hindered by the pharmacological interventions of mainstream medicine. However, homoeopathy's insistence that homoeopathic pharmaceuticals are necessary in aiding the vital force in restoring health places it in both camps and helps explain its appeal to various groups today as in the past.

Julia Green never abandoned the idea that homoeopathy would one day regain the popularity it enjoyed in the nineteenth century. With its institutional structure in ruins by the 1930s, Green still envisioned a future for the medical system to which she had dedicated her life. Highlighting the traditional link between healing and religion, she insisted that homoeopathy would flourish again "when this materialistic age has passed and a better, more spiritual one arrives."[27] Although few people consider today's society less materialistic than in previous decades, widespread interest in Eastern and Native American spiritual practices as well as the growth in religious fundamentalism in America reflects the appeal of the unseen, nonmaterial, metaphysical realm of life.

Because she was politically astute and eager for the American Foundation for Homoeopathy to succeed, Green downplayed the role of women—even relinquishing her position as chair of the board of trustees when the organization was criticized as a "ladies-only affair." Yet as Green was keenly aware, upon its introduction into the United States early in the nineteenth century, women were crucial to homoeopathy's success. Homoeopathy enjoyed its greatest surge in popularity in the nineteenth century in large part because it was associated with the cause of women's rights. After nearly disappearing in the middle decades of the twentieth century, homoeopathy was rejuvenated as part of the women's health movement of second wave feminism. As patients and members of lay leagues helping to popularize and sustain homoeopathy, and as professional and community leaders with successful medical practices, women were and are a vital force in homoeopathy's changing identity throughout the long course of its history.

Women in Homeopathic Medical Societies

This appendix shows the participation of women in local and national homeopathic medical societies. In addition to elected positions on executive boards, numerous women were appointed to specialty bureaus (committees), many serving as chairs, and were delegates to meetings of national societies. While not exhaustive, it shows the degree to which women held leadership positions in homeopathic professional organizations. The list was compiled in chronological order from various sources, including: Thomas Lindsley Bradford, *Bradford Scrapbooks: Biographies of Homoeopathic Physicians*, 35 vols. (1890–1918); Bradfords, *Biographies of Homoeopathic Physicians and Surgeons*, (Philadelphia 1918); William Harvey King, *A History of Homoeopathy and Its Institutions in America*, 4 vols. (New York and Chicago 1905); and other homeopathic journals, proceedings, and transactions of homeopathic medical societies.

1869   Zina Clements. Homoeopathic Medical Society of Northern New York, President

1873   Alice B. Campbell. Kings County Homoeopathic Medical Society, Corresponding Secretary

1874   Clara Yeomans. Iowa Homoeopathic Medical Society, Second Vice President

      J. A. Dunning. Homoeopathic Medical Society of Northwestern Pennsylvania, Vice President

      Corresta T. Canfield. Homoeopathic Medical Society of Northwestern Pennsylvania, Treasurer

1875   Elizabeth Avery. Kansas Homoeopathic Medical Society, Corresponding Secretary

1880   Millie J. Chapman. AIH, Chair, Bureau of Obstetrics
1881   Corresta T. Canfield. Homoeopathic Medical Society of the State of
        Pennsylvania, Board of Censors
1882   Maria Johnson. Homoeopathic Medical Society of the State of Penn-
        sylvania, Board of Censors
        Helena M. Cady. Pulaski County Homoeopathic Medical Society
        (Arkansas), Treasurer
1883   Maria Johnson. Homoeopathic Medical Society of the State of Penn-
        sylvania, Board of Censors
1884   Harriet Sartain. Homoeopathic Medical Society of the State of Penn-
        sylvania, Board of Censors
1886   Mary Branson. Homoeopathic Medical Society of the State of Penn-
        sylvania, Board of Censors
1889   Ada F. Bruce. Florida State Homoeopathic Medical Society, Vice
        President
1890   Sarah J. Milsop. Kentucky Homoeopathic Association, Chair, Bureau
        of Paedology
1891   Millie J. Chapman. Homoeopathic Medical Society of the State
        of Pennsylvania, Second Vice President; and Chair, Bureau of
        Gynecology
        Sarah J. Coe. Homoeopathic Medical Society of the State of Pennsyl-
        vania, Board of Censors
1892   Sarah J. Coe. Homoeopathic Medical Society of the State of Pennsyl-
        vania, Second Vice President
        Millie J. Chapman. AIH, Chair, Bureau of Paedology; Board of Cen-
        sors (thirty years)
1893   Julia Holmes Smith. World Congress of Homoeopathic Physicians and
        Surgeons, Vice President
        Millie J. Chapman. AIH, Second Vice President
        Amelia Burroughs. Homoeopathic Medical Society of Nebraska,
        President
        Sarah J. Coe. Homoeopathic Medical Society of the State of Pennsyl-
        vania, First Vice President
1894   Mary J. Safford (Blake). AIH, Board of Censors
        Corresta T. Canfield. AIH, Board of Censors
        Mary A. B. Wood. AIH, Board of Censors
        Julia Holmes Smith. AIH, Chair, Bureau of Obstetrics
        Millie J. Chapman. AIH, Second Vice President
        Eliza Lang McClure. Homoeopathic Medical Society of the State of
        Pennsylvania, Second Vice President

1895   Ella B. Goff. Homoeopathic Medical Society of the State of Pennsylvania, Chair, Bureau of Obstetrics

M. Margaret Hassler. Homoeopathic Medical Society of the State of Pennsylvania, Chair, Bureau of Paedology

Ella B. Goff. Homoeopathic Medical Society of the State of Pennsylvania, Board of Censors

Eliza Lang McClure. Homoeopathic Medical Society of the State of Pennsylvania, Board of Censors

Florence N. Saltonstall (Ward). California Homoeopathic Medical Society, Second Vice President

Eleanor F. Martin. California Homoeopathic Medical Society, Secretary

Lizzie Gray Gutherz. Southern Homoeopathic Medical Association, Corresponding Secretary

Clara Plimton. Southern Homoeopathic Medical Association, Chair, Bureau of Obstetrics

Emma F. A. Drake. Homoeopathic Medical Society of Colorado, Treasurer

Jane A. Walker. Homoeopathic Medical Society of Michigan, Chair, Bureau of Paedology

Julia M. Green. Homoeopathic Medical Society of Michigan, Chair, Bureau of Nervous Diseases

1896   Julia H. Smith. AIH, Board of Censors

Ida V. Stambach. California Homoeopathic Medical Society, Secretary; Chair, Bureau of Gynecology

Eleanor F. Martin. California Homoeopathic Medical Society, Treasurer

Susan Fenton. California Homoeopathic Medical Society, Chair, Bureau of Obstetrics

Lizzie Gray Gutherz. Southern Homoeopathic Medical Association, President

1897   Alice E. Rowe. Homoeopathic Medical Society of Western Massachusetts, Secretary

Nellie W. Stephenson. Lowell Hahnemann Club (Massachusetts), Secretary

Mary Florence Taft. IHA, Corresponding Secretary

1898   Alice Bush. California State Homoeopathic Society, Chair, Bureau of Anatomy, Physiology, and Pathology

Florence N. Ward. California Homoeopathic Medical Society, Chair, Gynecology

Eleanor F. Martin. California Homoeopathic Medical Society, Secretary (nine years)

1899   Sarah J. Millsop. AIH, Second Vice President
        Adelaide Lambert. Connecticut Homoeopathic Medical Society, Vice
        President
        Lucy Busenbark. Hahnemann Association of Iowa, Second Vice
        President
        Clarice J. Parsons. Allen Materia Medica Club of Springfield, Massa-
        chusetts, Secretary
        Susan M. Hicks. Southern Homoeopathic Association, Chair, Bureau
        of Paedology
        Martha A. Canfield. Homoeopathic Medical Society of Ohio, Chair,
        Bureau of Obstetrics
        Frances McMillan. Southern Homoeopathic Medical Association,
        Secretary
        Catherine H. Frank. Northern Indiana and Southern Michigan
        Homoeopathic Medical Association, Board of Censors

1900   Nancy Tiffany Williams. AIH, Second Vice President
        Sarah Guild-Leggett. IHA, Vice President
        Adelaide Lambert. Connecticut Homoeopathic Medical Society,
        President
        Ella B. Goff. Homoeopathic Medical Society of the State of Pennsyl-
        vania, Treasurer

1901   Florence N. Ward. IHA, Second Vice President
        Ella B. Goff. Homoeopathic Medical Society of the State of Pennsyl-
        vania, Treasurer

1903   M. Belle Brown. AIH, Second Vice President

1904   Sophia Penfield. Connecticut Homoeopathic Medical Society, President
        Mary Elizabeth Hanks. Homoeopathic Medical Society of Chicago,
        President
        Annie E. Spencer. AIH, Second Vice President

1906   Mary Elizabeth Hanks. Illinois Homoeopathic Medical Society,
        President
        Abby Janet Seymour. Erie County Homoeopathic Medical Society
        (Pennsylvania), President

1909   Ella Prentiss Upham. New Jersey Homoeopathic Medical Society,
        President

1910   Sarah M. Hobson. AIH, Second Vice President

1912   Carolyn Putnam. IHA, Vice President
        Clara Emerette Gary. AIH, Second Vice President

1913   Julia M. Green. IHA, Vice President
        Mary Elizabeth Hanks. AIH, Second Vice President

1914   Sarah M. Hobson. AIH, Secretary
         Anna D. Varner. AIH, Second Vice President
         Grace Hampton. IHA, Vice President
         Alice G. Henderson. Los Angeles County Homoeopathic Medical Society, Secretary
1915   Margaret Burgess Webster. IHA, Vice President
         Mary E. Mosher. AIH, Second Vice President
         Sarah M. Hobson. AIH, Secretary
         Julia H. Bass. Texas Homoeopathic Medical Association, Secretary
         Mary E. Glover. San Francisco County Homoeopathic Society, Secretary
         Mary Parker. Boston Society of Homoeopathy, Secretary
         Alice G. Henderson. Los Angeles County Homoeopathic Medical Society, Secretary
         Emily M. Luff. West Branch of the Chicago Homoeopathic Medical Society, Secretary
         Della MacMullen. Englewood Homoeopathic Medical Society (New Jersey), Secretary
         Elizabeth C. Maas. Northwestern Homoeopathic Medical Society, Secretary
         Mary E. Hopkins. Falls City Homoeopathic Medical Society of Louisville, Kentucky, Secretary
         Florence A. Richardson. Minneapolis Homoeopathic Medical Society, Secretary
         Sarah L. Guild-Leggett. Central New York Homoeopathic Medical Society, Secretary
         Margaret H. Schantz. Homoeopathic Medical Society of Berks County, Pennsylvania, Secretary
1916   Harriet Knudson Burnett. New Jersey State Homoeopathic Medical Society, Corresponding Secretary
1918   Florence N. Ward. AIH, Board of Trustees (three years)
1919   Harriet W. Hale. AIH, Second Vice President
         Anna Johnston. AIH, Board of Censors
1924   Gertrude K. Mack. AIH, Third Vice President
1925   Mary E. Hanks. AIH, Board of Trustees (three years)
1927   Florence E. Voorhees. AIH, Third Vice President
1928   Elizabeth Wright. IHA, Second Vice President
         Grace Stevens. IHA, Corresponding Secretary
         Julia M. Green. IHA, Necrologist
1930   Grace Stevens. IHA, President

Enumeration of Homeopathic and Regular Physicians, 1886, 1890–1893, and 1900

1886

| | Regulars | | Homeopaths | | Total |
	No.	%	No.	%	No.
Females					
Philadelphia	47	80	12	20	59
Boston	17	39	27	61	44
Chicago	36	39	56	61	92
New York	35	46	41	54	76
Males					
Philadelphia	1,427	86	235	14	1,662
Boston	706	86	116	14	822
Chicago	828	85	145	15	973
New York	1,848	91	183	9	2,031

1890/1893

| | Regulars | | Homeopaths | | Total |
	No.	%	No.	%	No.
Females					
Philadelphia	73	83	15	17	88
Boston	39	46	45	54	84
Chicago	64	40	95	60	159
New York	51	54	44	46	95
Brooklyn	13	28	34	72	47
Males					
Philadelphia	1,688	86	276	14	1,964
Boston	764	87	119	13	883
Chicago	1,495	80	382	20	1,877
New York	2,667	92	218	8	2,885
Brooklyn	956	87	149	13	1,105

1900

	Regulars		Homeopaths		Total
	No.	%	No.	%	No.
Females					
Philadelphia	109	80	28	20	137
Boston	65	49	69	51	134
Chicago	115	52	105	48	220
New York	90	61	58	39	148
Brooklyn	29	41	42	59	71
Males					
Philadelphia	1,683	82	375	18	2,058
Boston	570	82	126	18	696
Chicago	2,326	87	362	13	2,688
New York	3,387	94	229	6	3,616
Brooklyn	1,184	91	111	9	1,295

SOURCE: Numbers for the years 1886 and 1890 were hand counted from *The Medical and Surgical Directory of the United States* (Detroit: R.L. Polk); and the years 1893 and 1900 from *The Medical and Surgical Register of the United States and Canada* (Detroit: R.L. Polk). Percentages throughout Appendix B are calculated individually for each city and within the Female and Male categories. "Total" refers to homeopathic and regular physicians only, versus the entire practitioner population in each city. According to William Rothstein's estimates, homeopaths comprised about 8 percent of all practitioners listed in Polk's *Register* (1898). In 1900, there were approximately 110,000 regular physicians, 10,000 homeopaths, and over 10,000 practitioners combined in all other modalities nationwide. Thus, homeopaths comprised 9 percent of the regular/homeopathic total. See William G. Rothstein, *American Physicians in the Nineteenth Century: From Sects to Science* (Baltimore: Johns Hopkins University Press, 1985) 344–345. Figures for Boston are from the 1893 *Register*; and those for Philadelphia, New York, and Brooklyn are from the *Register* of 1900.

Notes

Introduction   Homeopathy as "Other"

1. Thomas C. Harbaugh, ed., *Centennial History: Troy, Piqua, and Miami County, Ohio and Representative Citizens* (Chicago: Richmond-Arnold Publishing Co., 1909).

2. See, for example Mary Roth Walsh, *"Doctors Wanted: No Women Need Apply": Sexual Barriers in the Medical Profession, 1835–1975* (New Haven: Yale University Press, 1977); Regina Morantz-Sanchez, *Sympathy and Science: Women Physicians in American Medicine* (New York: Oxford University Press, 1985); Ruth J. Abram, ed., *"Send Us a Lady Physician": Women Doctors in America, 1835–1920* (New York: W. W. Norton & Co., 1985); Gloria Moldow, *Women Doctors in Gilded-Age Washington: Race, Gender, and Professionalization* (Urbana and Chicago: University of Illinois Press, 1987); Thomas Neville Bonner, *To the Ends of the Earth: Women's Search for Education in Medicine* (Cambridge: Harvard University Press, 1992); Ellen Singer More and Maureen A. Milligan, eds., *The Empathic Practitioner: Empathy, Gender, and Medicine* (New Brunswick, N.J.: Rutgers University Press, 1994); and Ellen Singer More, *Restoring the Balance: Women Physicians and the Profession of Medicine, 1850–1995* (Cambridge: Harvard University Press, 1999).

3. For an excellent overview of the subject, see Naomi Rogers, "Women and Sectarian Medicine," in *Women, Health, and Medicine in America: A Historical Handbook* (New York: Garland Press, 1990), 273–302. More particularized studies include: Susan Cayleff, *Wash and Be Healed: The Water-Cure Movement and Women's Health* (Philadelphia: Temple University Press, 1987); Jane Donegan, *"Hydropathic Highway to Health": Women and Water-Cure in Ante-bellum America* (Westport, Conn.: Greenwood Press, 1986); Ronald L. Numbers, *Prophetess of Health: Ellen G. White and the Origins of Seventh-Day Adventist Health Reform* (Knoxville: University of Tennessee Press, 1992); Jonathan Butler and Rennie B. Schoepflin, "Charismatic Women and Health: Mary Baker Eddy, Ellen G. White, and Aimee Semple McPherson," in *Women, Health, and Medicine in America*, 329–357.

4. While the homeopathic system was based on the "law of similars" or "like cures like," the term "allopathy" is from the Greek, alloison pathos, meaning "heterogeneous" or "unlike" disease. According to Hahnemann, allopaths prescribed on the basis of the Galenic theory of contraria contrarii, the opposite of "like cures like." Although regular physicians argued it was an inaccurate description of their therapeutic practices, the term was widely adopted by nonorthodox groups. See Naomi Rogers, *An Alternative Path: The Making and Remaking of Hahnemann Medical College and Hospital of Philadelphia* (New Brunswick, N.J.: Rutgers University Press,

1998), 7; and Harris L. Coulter, *Divided Legacy: The Conflict Between Homoeopathy and the American Medical Association,* 2d ed. (Berkeley, Calif.: North Atlantic Books, 1982), viii.

5. See John Harley Warner, "Orthodoxy and Otherness: Homeopathy and Regular Medicine in Nineteenth-Century America," in *Culture, Knowledge, and, Healing: Historical Perspectives of Homeopathic Medicine in Europe and North America,* ed. Robert Jutte, Guenter B. Risse, and John Woodward (Sheffield, UK: European Association for the History of Medicine and Health Publications 1998), 5–29.

6. Mary J. Safford (Blake) to the New York Medical College and Hospital for Women Alumnae Association, n.d., Boston, Minutes of the NYMCHW Alumnae Association, 1879.

7. Sophia Penfield to NYMCHW Alumnae Association, 23 March 1878, Minutes of the NYMCHW Alumnae Association, 1879. Danbury, Conn.

8. Samuel Augustus Fisk to Dr. William Williamson, 26 September 1875, Massachusetts Medical Society Collection, 3–4, Northampton, Mass.

9. *2000 Membership Directory & Homeopathic Resource Guide* (Alexandria, Va.: National Center for Homeopathy, 2000).

10. Lauren Fox, RNCS, FNP, interview by author, Falmouth, Mass., 3 November 1994; Maesimund B. Panos, M.D., interview by author, Tipp City, Ohio, 10 March 1996. Although "holism" in medicine has multiple meanings and is, perhaps, not a particularly useful term because of its imprecision, it is often used by advocates today in describing the appeal of homeopathy. Within this context, its definition is closely related to "organismic holism" described by Charles Rosenberg, i.e., the body as an integrated functioning system, transcending the individual parts and processes making up that system, influenced by "an intrinsic and almost mystical wisdom of the body." See Charles E. Rosenberg, "Holism in Twentieth-Century Medicine," in *Greater than the Parts: Holism in Biomedicine, 1920–1950,* ed. Christopher Lawrence and George Weisz (New York: Oxford University Press, 1998), 339.

11. In the interview with author on 3 November 1994, Fox estimates her practice is 70 percent adult women.

12. National Center for Homeopathy, *1998 Directory: Practitioners, Study Groups, Pharmacies, Resources,* (Alexandria, Va.: National Center for Homeopathy 1998). Among the 476 practitioners listed in the directory, approximately 182 are women in various professions including: nursing, nurse practitioner, M.D., physician assistant, chiropractor, veterinarian, and licensed or certified acupuncturist, nutritionist, and midwife.

Chapter 1 The New School of Medicine

1. For concise descriptions of homeopathy's introduction and dissemination in the United States, see Martin Kaufman, *Homeopathy in America: The Rise and Fall of a Medical Heresy* (Baltimore: Johns Hopkins University Press, 1971); and Harris L. Coulter, *Divided Legacy: The Conflict Between Homoeopathy and the American Medical Association, Science and Ethics in American Medicine, 1800–1914,* 2d ed. (Berkeley, Calif.: North Atlantic Books, 1982), 101–111.

2. Naomi Rogers, *An Alternative Path: The Making and Remaking of Hahnemann Medical College and Hospital of Philadelphia* (New Brunswick, N.J.: Rutgers University Press, 1998), 4.

3. These figures are from William G. Rothstein, *American Physicians in the Nineteenth Century: From Sects to Science* (Baltimore: Johns Hopkins University Press, 1985). See Appendix 4, "Enumerations of Physicians, 1850–1900," 344–345.

4. G. W. Bailey, M.D., "A Plea for the Children," *Hahnemannian Monthly* 3, no. 11 (November 1881): 653.
5. In comparison, women graduates of regular medical colleges numbered 648 in the year 1890 alone, and by 1900 there were roughly seven thousand women physicians, including homeopaths. However, women regulars comprised a smaller percentage of their profession (4 to 5 percent in the last decade of the century.) See, Regina Morantz-Sanchez, *Sympathy and Science: Women Physicians in American Medicine* (New York: Oxford University Press, 1985), 92, 249. I am extremely grateful to Julian Winston of the National Center for Homeopathy for providing me with the names of 25,000 women he compiled into a database of homeopathic physicians: *American Homeopaths: 1825–1963* (Tawa, NZ: Great Auk Publishing), hereafter referred to as Winston Database.
6. Charles E. Rosenberg and John Harley Warner have been instrumental in making this point about science. See Charles E. Rosenberg, "Introduction: Science, Society, and Social Thought," in *No Other Gods: On Science and American Social Thought* (Baltimore: Johns Hopkins University Press, 1976), 1–21; and John Harley Warner, *The Therapeutic Perspective: Medical Practice, Knowledge, and Identity in America, 1820–1885* (Cambridge: Harvard University Press, 1986); "Science in Medicine," *OSIRIS* 2, no. 1 (1985): 37–58; and "The Therapeutic Revolution: Medicine, Meaning, and Social Change in Nineteenth-Century America," *Perspectives in Biology and Medicine* 20 (1977): 485–506.
7. William G. Rothstein, "The Botanical Movements and Orthodox Medicine," in *Other Healers: Unorthodox Medicine in America*, ed. Norman Gevitz (Baltimore: Johns Hopkins University Press, 1988), 29–51; and Susan E. Cayleff, "Gender, Ideology, and the Water-Cure Movement," in *Other Healers: Unorthodox Medicine in America*, ed. Norman Gevitz (Baltimore: Johns Hopkins University Press, 1988), 82–98.
8. Humoralism was the theoretical underpinning for understanding the cause of disease since Hippocratic times. The proper balance of humors or fluids of blood, black bile, yellow bile, and phlegm were active agents whose proper balance and regulation was necessary for curing disease and maintaining health. See W. F. Bynum, *Science and the Practice of Medicine in the Nineteenth Century* (Cambridge: Cambridge University Press, 1994), 13, 30; and Roy Porter, *The Greatest Benefit to Mankind: A Medical History of Humanity* (New York: W. W. Norton & Co., 1997), 246.
9. Porter, *Greatest Benefit to Mankind*, 260–262.
10. Ibid., 17–18.
11. Rogers, *An Alternative Path*, 5. The term homeopathy means "like-suffering," derived from the Greek *homoios pathos*.
12. Renate Wittern, "The Origins of Homoeopathy in Germany," *Clio Medica* 22, (1991): 52.
13. Richard Haehl, *Samuel Hahnemann: His Life and Work* 1, (1923; reprint, New Delhi: B. Jain Publishers, 1995), 37 (page citations are to the reprint edition).
14. This essay first appeared in *The Journal for Practicing Physicians* in 1796. One physician noted that Hahnemann originally used the subjunctive form of the verb *curo* or *Curentur*, which in *Similia Similibus Curentur* is translated "Let likes be treated by likes." In translations the verb was changed to the indicative form, Similia Similibus Curantor, meaning "Likes cures Likes." Hahnemann was apparently annoyed at this alteration. See J. H. McClelland, "Curentur or Curantur?" *Transactions of the AIH* (n.p., 1899): 99–101.
15. John Harley Warner, "Orthodoxy and Otherness: Homeopathy and Regular Medicine in Nineteenth-Century America," in *Culture, Knowledge, and Healing: Historical Perspectives of Homeopathic Medicine in Europe and North America* ed. Robert

Jutte, Guenter B. Risse, and John Woodward (Sheffield, UK: European Association for the History of Medicine and Health Publications, 1998), 7; and Wittern, "The Origins of Homoeopathy in Germany," 59.

16. Samuel Hahnemann, *Organon of Medicine*, 5th & 6th ed., rev. and enl., trans. William Boericke (1810; reprint, New Delhi: B. Jain Publishers, 1996), 32–34.

17. Rogers, *An Alternative Path*, 6.

18. Hahnemann, *Organon of Medicine*, 5th & 6th ed., 144.

19. Ibid., 26–27, 29.

20. Carroll Dunham, "*Lilium-tigrinum*—A Summary of a Few Provings upon Women," *North American Journal of Homoeopathy* 1, no. 11 (November 1870): 160.

21. Hahnemann, *Organon of Medicine*, 5th ed., 101.

22. Ibid., 171.

23. Wittern, "The Origins of Homoeopathy in Germany," 56.

24. Hahnemann's doctrine of psora may have been a variation on Greek theories positing that open, suppurating wounds conveyed poisoned blood out of the body.

25. Rogers, *An Alternative Path*, 4; and Coulter, *Divided Legacy*, 101–102. Constantine Hering's *The Homoeopathist or Domestic Physician* was published in two volumes from 1835 to 1838 by J. G. Wesselhoeft, Philadelphia; *Condensed Materia Medica* was published by Boericke and Tafel, Philadelphia (1877).

26. William Harvey King, ed., *History of Homoeopathy and Its Institutions* 3 (New York and Chicago: Lewis Publishing Co., 1905), 19; and Josef M. Schmidt, "Homeopathy in the American West: Its German Connections," in *Culture, Knowledge, and Healing*, 139–172.

27. Rogers, *An Alternative Path*, 15.

28. Warner, *The Therapeutic Perspective*, 5, 85. Note especially Chapter 3, "The Principle of Specificity," 58–80. Warner points out that practice according to specificity, i.e., prescribing according to an individual's unique circumstances and characteristics, was an essential part of regular physicians' identities, distinguishing them from quacks. Regular physicians claimed homeopaths routinely prescribed uniform therapy for those classified with the same ailment. This was, of course, exactly the criticism lodged by homeopaths against regulars. Warner cites lecture notes of homeopathic students which, he said, resemble cookbooks, listing fixed recipes for each disease. It is likely that both groups of physicians favored certain drugs for commonly encountered, recognizable disease states. In her lecture notebook dated 1863–1864 from the New York Medical College and Hospital for Women, Anna Manning Comfort notes that "Thuja [arbor vitae] given Homeopathically is almost a specific for varioloia (sic) & small pox." Use of the term "specific" in this sense had a negative connotation, implying that treatment was not individualized to a patient's needs but rather matched to a named disease. From Comfort Family Papers, *Extracts from Mrs. Dr. Loziers Lectures* box 14, Syracuse University Archives.

29. *Ten Reasons for Preferring Homoeopathy to the Common System of Medical Treatment, By the Father of a Family* Philadelphia: College of Physicians of Philadelphia, CPP pamphlet 168.

30. James H. Cassedy, *American Medicine and Statistical Thinking, 1800–1860* (Cambridge: Harvard University Press, 1984), 125. Sir Francis Bacon is linked with a quantitative approach to science beginning at the turn of the eighteenth century when rational decision-making was based on inductions from massive amounts of data.

31. Constantine Hering, introductory course lecture, Philadelphia, 1867–1868 (Hahnemann College, 1868).

32. Hahnemann, *Organon of Medicine*, 6th ed., 111–112; *Organon of Medicine*, 5th ed., 217–218.

33. Hering, *The Homoeopathic Domestic Physician*, 9 ed. (Philadelphia: Hahnemann Publishing House, 1883), 326–327.
34. E. B. Nash, *How to Take the Case and Find the Simillimum* (reprint, New Delhi: B. Jain Publishers n.d.).
35. Guy Beckley Stearns, "Case Taking," Homeopathy 3 (July 1921; reprint, CPP pamphlet, American Institute of Homeopathy).
36. Dr. James Tyler Kent, *What the Doctor Needs to Know in Order to Make a Successful Prescription* (reprint, Calcutta: P. K. Ghosh, 1957), 5.
37. Elizabeth Stuart Phelps, *Avis* (1877), 300, as cited in Christine Stansell, "Elizabeth Stuart Phelps: A Study in Female Rebellion," *Massachusetts Review* 13 (1979): 249.
38. See for example, Steven M. Stowe, "Seeing Themselves at Work: Physicians and the Case Narrative in the Mid-Nineteenth-Century American South," *American Historical Review* 101, no.1 (February 1996): 41–79.
39. Virginia G. Drachman, "Women Doctors and the Women's Medical Movement: Feminism and Medicine, 1850–1895" (Ph.D. diss., State University of New York at Buffalo, 1976).
40. D. W. Cathell, *The Physician Himself and What He Should Add to His Scientific Acquirements* (1882), 141, cited in Drachman dissertation, 22.
41. Carroll Dunham, M.D., *Homoeopathy the Science of Therapeutics: A Collection of Papers Elucidating and Illustrating the Principles of Homoeopathy* (1877; reprint, New Delhi: B. Jain Publishers, 1997), 89–91.
42. Conrad Wesselhoeft, M.D., "Some Observations on Neurasthenia and its Treatment," in *Transactions of the World's Homoeopathic Congress* (1893): 784.
43. Julia Minerva Green, "Dealing With Our Patients," in *Proceedings of the International Hahnemannian Association* (1912): 55.
44. The work of John Harley Warner has been an important addition to the extensive literature on the influence of the Paris School on American medicine. See "Remembering Paris: Memory and the American Disciples of French Medicine in the Nineteenth Century," *Bulletin of the History of Medicine* 65 (1991): 301–325; and *Against the Spirit of System: The French Impulse in Nineteenth-Century American Medicine* (Princeton: Princeton University Press, 1998). Classic studies on the birth and growth of the clinic and the emergence of Paris as the most influential center of Western medicine include: Erwin H. Ackernecht, *Medicine at the Paris Hospital, 1794–1848* (Baltimore: Johns Hopkins University Press, 1967); and Michel Foucault, *The Birth of the Clinic: An Archeology of Medical Perceptions*, trans. A. M. Sheridan (New York: Pantheon Books, 1973).
45. John Harley Warner, "The Fall and Rise of Professional Mystery: Epistemology, Authority, and the Emergence of Laboratory Medicine in Nineteenth-Century America," in *The Laboratory Revolution in Medicine*, ed. Andrew Cunningham and Perry Williams (Cambridge: Cambridge University Press, 1992), 120–121.
46. John Harley Warner, *Against the Spirit of System: The French Impulse in Nineteenth-Century American Medicine* (Princeton: Princeton University Press, 1998), 250.
47. Ibid., 172; and W. C. Smith, "Remarks on Empiricism" (M.D. thesis, Medical University of the State of South Carolina, 1850), cited in John Harley Warner, "Orthodoxy and Otherness," 14, f 44. See also, Cunningham and Williams, "Introduction," in *The Laboratory Revolution in Medicine*, 2.
48. Warner, "Orthodoxy and Otherness," 12–13.
49. Ibid., 15.
50. Kaufman, *Homeopathy in America*, 53.
51. Rogers, *An Alternative Path*, 27. See also King, "The Western College of Homoeopathic Medicine," in *History of Homoeopathy* 3 (1905): 14; and "Hahnemann Medical College of Chicago," *History of Homeopathy* 2: 341.

52. Although Hahnemann's *Materia Medica Pura*, trans. C. J. Hempel (New York: W. Radden, 1846) was widely used, several multivolume materia medicas were published in the nineteenth century. Timothy Field Allen edited *The Encyclopaedia of Pure Materia Medica*, whose ten volumes were published from 1874 to 1879. The eight-volume *Cyclopaedia of Drug Pathogenesy* (1885), ed. Richard Hugues and J. P. Dake, was issued under the combined auspices of the British Homoeopathic Society and the AIH. Another widely used materia medica was that of Constantine Hering. Building on Adolph Lippe's *Text-Book of Materia Medica* (1866), Hering's *The Guiding Symptoms of the Materia Medica* was published in ten volumes beginning in 1878 and ending in 1891.

53. James Blakely, M.D., "Report of the Committee on Drug Provings and New Remedies," *Transactions of the Homoeopathic Medical Society of the State of Pennsylvania*, 1866–1867: 59.

54. *Transactions of the AIH*, 1874: 267.

55. *Transactions of the World Homeopathic Convention*, 1876: 263, 267.

56. Dunham, "Lilium-tigrinum—A Summary of a Few Provings Upon Women," *North American Journal of Homoeopathy 1*, no. 11 (November 1870): 160.

57. Ruben Ludlam, M.D., *Medical and Surgical Lectures on the Diseases of Women: A Clinical and Systematic Treatise*, 5th ed. rev. (Chicago: Duncan Bros., 1881), 160.

58. Morantz-Sanchez, *Sympathy and Science*, 70; and "The Gendering of Empathic Expertise: How Women Physicians Became More Empathic than Men," in *The Empathic Practitioner: Empathy, Gender, and Medicine*, ed. Ellen Singer More and Maureen A. Milligan (New Brunswick, N.J.: Rutgers University Press, 1994), 40–58. See also, Ellen Singer More, "'Empathy' Enters the Profession of Medicine," in *The Empathic Practitioner*, 19–39.

59. Warner, *Against the Spirit of System*, 282.

60. Warner, *The Therapeutic Perspective*, 243–245, 253.

61. Kaufman, *Homeopathy in America*, 129.

62. Naomi Rogers, "American Homeopathy Confronts Scientific Medicine," in *Culture, Knowledge, and Healing: Historical Perspectives of Homeopathic Medicine in Europe and North America*, ed. Robert Jutte, Guenter B. Risse, and John Woodward (Sheffield, UK: European Association for the History of Medicine and Health Publications, 1998), 35.

63. W. E. Payne, "Miscellaneous Items," *North American Journal of Homoeopathy* 1.3 (February 1871): 430. Hahnemannians typically employed high-potency single remedies and internal remedies rather than topical medications.

64. Carroll Dunham, "Liberty of Medical Opinion and Action: A Vital Necessity and a Great Responsibility," *Transactions of the Homoeopathic Medical Society of the State of New York* 8 (1870).

65. Ibid., 738.

66. Ibid., 741.

67. C. Pearson, "History of the Society," *Proceedings of the IHA 1881–1883*: 5–9.

68. Adolph Lippe, "The Secession Movement in Medicine," *The United States Medical Investigator* 6, no. 8 (October 15, 1877): 495.

69. Meaning Hahnemannian homeopathy.

70. *Proceedings of the IHA* (1887): 217–221.

71. Frederick P. Henry, ed., *Founders' Week Memorial Volume* (Philadelphia: City of Philadelphia Commemoration of the Two Hundred and Twenty-fifth Anniversary of its Founding, 1909), 710–712, 181–182.

72. Figures are from the second Annual Report of the Women's Homoeopathic Association of Pennsylvania (1885).

73. According to the fourth Annual Report of the Medical, Surgical, and Maternity Hospitals of the Women's Homoeopathic Association of Pennsylvania (1886), the physicians were Almah J. Frisby, Jennie Medley, Harriet S. French, Harriet Judd Sartain, Lora Jackson, Mary Branson, Josephine Van Deusen, Eliza Lang McClure, Emma T. Schreiner, Eliza Pettingill, and Anna M. Marshall.

74. Adolph Lippe, "The Hospitals of the Women's Homoeopathic Association of Pennsylvania," *The Homoeopathic Physician* 7 (May 1887): 178.

75. *Proceedings of the IHA* (1887): 218.

76. According to William Kirtsos, collector of antiquarian homeopathic literature, *The Hahnemannian* began as a vehicle for strict homeopathy. However, after the sixth volume, it no longer represented the views of that group.

77. *Hahnemannian Monthly* 22, no. 5 (May 1887): 304–305.

78. Rogers, *An Alternative Path*, 68–73.

79. Lippe, "The Hospitals of the Woman's Homoeopathic Association of Pennsylvania," 216–217.

80. See David Rosner, *A Once Charitable Enterprise* (Princeton: Princeton University Press, 1987); and Morris Vogel, *The Invention of the Modern Hospital: Boston, 1870–1930* (Chicago: Chicago University Press, 1980).

81. Warner, *The Therapeutic Perspective*, 5, 120.

82. Rogers, "American Homeopathy Confronts Scientific Medicine," 46.

83. IHA members in 1910 included 138 men and 34 women. The AIH listed 309 women out of a total of 2,512 members. Data hand counted from *Proceedings of the IHA* (1910) and the *International Homoeopathic Medical Directory*, 1911–1912. Estimates on the percentage of women in the profession in 1910 are based on the number of women (1,020) among all graduates of homeopathic colleges (6,300) between 1890 and 1905.

Chapter 2 The Choice of Homeopathy

1. Active in his new-found profession, Bayard was one of the first members of the American Institute of Homoeopathy and a founding member of the IHA in 1881, earning a reputation as one of New York's foremost Hahnemannian physicians. See Christopher Ellithorp, "Elizabeth Cady Stanton" in *The American Homeopath* 3 (1997): 103–105.

2. Lois W. Banner, *Elizabeth Cady Stanton: A Radical for Woman's Rights* (Boston: Little, Brown & Co., 1980), 50, 69–70.

3. Elizabeth Cady Stanton to Lucretia Mott, 22 October 1852, in *The Oven Birds: American Women on Womanhood, 1820–1920*, ed. Gail Parker (Garden City, N.Y.: Anchor Books, 1972), 260.

4. Naomi Rogers, "American Homeopathy Confronts Scientific Medicine," in *Culture, Knowledge, and Healing: Historical Perspectives of Homeopathic Medicine in Europe and North America*, ed. Robert Jutte, Guenter B. Risse, and John Woodward (Sheffield, UK: European Association for the History of Medicine and Health Publications, 1998), 37.

5. Sydney E. Ahlstrom, *A Religious History of the American People* (New Haven: Yale University Press, 1972), 475.

6. Robert C. Fuller, *Alternative Medicine and American Religious Life* (New York: Oxford University Press, 1989), 25, 56.

7. Regina Markell Morantz, "Making Women Modern: Middle-Class Women and Health Reform in America," in *Women and Health in America*, ed. Judith Walzer Leavitt (Madison: University of Wisconsin Press, 1984), 346–358; Martha Verbrugge, *Able-Bodied Womanhood: Personal Health and Social Change in Nineteenth-*

Century Boston (New York: Oxford University Press, 1988), 26. Scholars have placed women's interest in water-cure therapeutics at mid-century within the context of social egalitarianism, the glorification of the individual in literature and philosophy, a lessening of the hold of established religions, and a heightened emphasis on participation in the political process. See Susan Cayleff, *Wash and Be Healed: The Water-Cure Movement and Women's Health* (Philadelphia: Temple University Press, 1987); and Jean L. Silver-Isenstadt, *Shameless: the Visionary Life of Mary Gove Nichols* (Baltimore: Johns Hopkins University Press, 2002).

8. Elizabeth P. Peabody, "Memorial of William Wesselhoeft, 1859," in *The Pioneers of Homoeopathy* (Philadelphia: Boericke & Tafel, 1897), 658–659.

9. Elizabeth Young, "A Wound of One's Own: Louisa May Alcott's Civil War Fiction," *American Quarterly* 48, no. 3 (September 1996): 439–474.

10. Louisa M. Alcott, *Jo's Boys and How They Turned Out: A Sequel to Little Men* (Boston: Little, Brown & Co., 1925).

11. Charles A. Lee, "Homoeopathy," *The New Church Messenger* 1, no. 23 (1 February 1854), 365.

12. Fuller, *Alternative Medicine and American Religious Life*, 51 486.

13. Joel Myerson, Daniel Shealy, and Madeleine B. Stern, eds., *The Selected Letters of Louisa May Alcott* (Boston and Toronto: Little, Brown & Co., 1987), 196–197.

14. Julian Winston, *The Faces of Homoeopathy: An Illustrated History of the First 200 Years* (Tawa, NZ: Great Awk Publishing, 1999)

15. Julian Winston, "Kent: A Modern Biography of James Tyler Kent," *The American Homeopath* 2 (Summer 1995): 9.

16. Ronald L. Numbers, "Do-It-Yourself the Sectarian Way," in *"Send Us a Lady Physician" Women Doctors in America, 1835–1920*, ed. Ruth J. Abram (New York: W. W. Norton & Co., 1985), 43–54.

17. Constantine Hering, *Domestic Physician*, 233 cited in Harris L. Coulter, *Divided Legacy: The Conflict between Homoeopathy and the American Medical Association Science and Ethics in American Medicine, 1800–1914*, 2d ed. (Berkeley: North Atlantic Books, 1982), 115.

18. Joseph Hooper, M.D., "Homeopathy: What are its Claims on Public Confidence?," CPP pamphlet *Homoeopathy* 169, 6.

19. Numbers, "Do-It-Yourself the Sectarian Way," 48.

20. *North American Journal of Homoeopathy* 1, no. 11 (November 1870): 280.

21. Numbers, "Do-It-Yourself the Sectarian Way," 48.

22. Rita Dunlevy, "Paper Read Before the Alumnae Association of the New York Medical College and Hospital for Women," *Cresset* 10, no. 2 (December 1906), 5.

23. Comparisons are based on characteristics of regular women physicians noted by Regina Morantz-Sanchez in *Sympathy and Science: Women Physicians in American Medicine* (New York: Oxford University Press, 1985); and those of approximately two hundred women homeopaths from the following sources: William Harvey King, *History of Homoeopathy*, 1–4; Egbert Cleave, *Biographical Cyclopaedia of Homoeopathic Physicians and Surgeons*; Thomas Lindsley Bradford, *American Homoeopathic Biographic Cyclopaedia of Homoeopathic Physicians and Surgeons*; and *Bradford Scrapbooks: Biographies of Homoeopathic Physicians* (thirty-five scrapbooks compiled by Bradford during his tenure as librarian at Hahnemann Medical College in Philadelphia, 1890–1918); published proceedings of national, state, and local homeopathic medical societies; and manuscript material in university and historical society archives.

24. *Biographical Cyclopaedia of Homoeopathic Physicians and Surgeons*, ed., s.v. "Reid."

25. *Biographical Cyclopaedia*, ed., s.v. "Chase."

26. "Dr. M. Belle Brown," *Cresset* 9, no. 7 (June 1906), 9–10; and J. C. Hover, et al., *Memories of the Miami Valley* 1 (Chicago: Robert O. Law Co., 1919), 106.

27. Andrew Sartain to Samuel Sartain, Connecticut, 20 July 1854, Sartain Collection, Historical Society of Pennsylvania.

28. Hamilton Willcox, "Eulogy," (read at a meeting of the Ladies' Suffrage Committee, New York City, 2 May 1888).

29. Nancy F. Cott, *The Grounding of Modern Feminism* (New Haven: Yale University Press, 1987), 3, 16–17.

30. Morantz-Sanchez, *Sympathy and Science*, 50, 56, 135–137.

31. Anna Manning Comfort, "Life Sketch of Anna Manning Comfort, M.D.," (1931) American Medical Women's Association Historical Collection.

32. Seventy-six women were involved in the study. Almost three-quarters had annual incomes ranging from $1,000 to $4,000. See Emily F. Pope, Emma L. Call, and C. Augusta Pope, *The Practice of Medicine by Women in the United States* (Boston: 1881), in Mary Roth Walsh, *Doctors Wanted No Women Need Apply: Sexual Barriers in the Medical Profession, 1835–1975* (New Haven: Yale University Press, 1977), 184.

33. Harriet Judd Sartain to Samuel Sartain 5 July 1854, Sartain Collection, Historical Society of Pennsylvania.

34. Frances Janney Derby to Anne Janney Deming, 14 October 1877, Janney Family Papers, MSS 142, Ohio Historical Society.

35. Frances Janney Derby to Rebecca Smith Janney, 28 October 1877, Janney Family Papers, MSS 142, Ohio Historical Society.

36. Morantz-Sanchez, *Sympathy and Science*, 73; and Naomi Rogers, "Women and Sectarian Medicine," in *Women, Health, and Medicine in America: A Historical Handbook*, ed. Rima D. Apple (New Brunswick, N.J.: Rutgers University Press, 1992), 291.

37. While the first catalog of the NYMCHW claimed the instituion was "wholly non-sectarian," lectures on homeopathic materia medica were part of the school's curriculum from the beginning. Two years later it was identified in the annual catalog as a homeopathic medical college. See Anna Manning Comfort Lectures, Comfort Family Papers, box 14, Syracuse University Archives.

38. Male physicians who supported Lozier included regular physicians Drs. Jacoby and Janeway, and homeopath William Todd Helmuth. See Bertha L. Selmon, "The New York Medical College and Hospital for Women," *Medical Woman's Journal* (April 1946): 44.

39. *The Revolution* 2, no. 23 (10 December 1868): 361.

40. See *Papers of Elizabeth Cady Stanton and Susan B. Anthony* (Wilmington, Del.: Scholarly Resources, 1991), microfilm reel 1: 42, 82, 169–170, 283, 295, 331; reel 5: 37–38; reel 18: 866–869.

41. *Proceedings of the International Hahnemannian Association*, 1909: 5.

42. Alice B. Campbell, M.D., "The Woman Doctor—Her Achievements and Her Disabilities," *Cresset* 1, no. 2 (December 1897): 17–19. Unfortunately, the record of this case is missing from the archives of the New York State Library in Albany.

43. Morantz-Sanchez, *Sympathy and Science*, 71.

44. Rogers, "Women and Sectarian Medicine," 273–302.

45. Gloria Moldow, *Women Doctors in Gilded-Age Washington: Race, Gender, and Professionalization* (Urbana and Chicago: University of Illinois Press, 1987), 17, 23, 135–137.

46. Sarah Deutsch, "Learning to Talk More Like a Man: Boston Women's Class-Bridging Organization, 1870–1940," *American Historical Review* 97, no. 2 (April 1992): 383.

47. Harriet Clisby, "Some Reminisences of Australia and America," WEIU Collection, 124–127.

48. Cott, *The Grounding of Modern Feminism*, 17.

49. Deutsch, "Learning to Talk More Like a Man," 388.

50. *Bradford Scrapbooks* vol. 27; and Mary Safford to James Jackson Putnam, Breslau,

Poland, 16 April 1871, Women in Medicine Collection, MS/c 4.2, Francis A. Countway Library of Medicine.

51. Frances Janney Derby to Rebecca Smith Janney, 23 May 1875, and 9 June 1875, Janney Family Papers, MSS 142, Ohio Historical Society.

52. Abba Goold Woolsoon, ed., *Dress Reform: On Dress as it Affects the Health of Women* (Boston: Roberts Brothers, 1874).

53. Susan Shifrin, "From the kingdom of fancy, fashion and foolery, to the kingdom of reason and righteousness . . . : Dress Reform and the Constraints of Clothing on Women Physicians at the Woman's Medical College of Pennsylvania, 1850–1900," In *Collections: The Newsletter of the Archives and Special Collections on Women in Medicine* 27 (October 1993), 5.

54. Woolsoon, ed., *Dress Reform*, 7, 92.

55. Ibid., 91.

56. Ibid.

57. William A. Linkugel and Martha Solomon, *Anna Howard Shaw: Suffrage Orator and Social Reformer* (Westport, Conn.: Greenwood Press, 1991), 8.

58. Winton U. Solberg, "Martha G. Ripley: Pioneer Doctor and Social Reformer," *Minnesota History* 39, no. 1, (spring 1964): 26.

59. Ibid., 12–17.

60. Harris L. Coulter, *Divided Legacy: The Conflict Between Homeopathy and the American Medical Association, Science, and Ethics in American Medicine, 1800–1914*, 2d ed. (Berkeley, Calif.: North Atlantic Books, 1982); Martin Kaufman, *Homeopathy in America: The Rise and Fall of a Medical Heresy* (Baltimore and London: Johns Hopkins University Press, 1971); and Phillip A. Nicholls, *Homeopathy and the Medical Profession* (London: Croom Helm, 1988).

61. Michael P. Duffy, "A Progression of Sectarianism: Homeopathy in Massachusetts from 1855 to 1875" (bachelor's thesis, Harvard University, 1982).

62. Names provided by Barbara Williams, archivist, Hahnemann University.

63. Edward C. Atwater, "The Physicians of Rochester, New York, 1860–1910: A Study in Professional History 2," *Bulletin of the History of Medicine* 51 (1977): 99.

64. Eliza J. Merrick, M.D. to Dr. Elizabeth Mason-Hohl, 30 October 1945; and "Stella Manning Perkins: A Reminiscence," by Ellen Perkins Doane, Alumnae Files, Archives and Special Collections on Women in Medicine and Homeopathy, Drexel University.

65. *Scrapbook*, Comfort Family Papers.

66. Rothstein based his estimate on data in R. L. Polk, ed., *Medical and Surgical Register of the United States* (1898). This estimate is reinforced by the number of homeopathic medical school graduates in the years 1890, 1900, and 1903—also about 8 percent. See William Rothstein, *American Physicians in the nineteenth Century: From Sects to Science* (Baltimore: Johns Hopkins University Press, 1985), 345.

67. *Brooklyn Daily Eagle* 29 March 1870, 7, cited in William Seraile, "Susan McKinney Steward: New York State's First African-American Woman Physician," *Afro-Americans in New York Life and History* 9, no. 2 (1985), 31.

68. Seraile, "Susan McKinney Steward," 27–28, 30.

69. Seraile, "Susan McKinney Steward," 34.

70. "Wealthy Negro Citizens," *New York Times*, 14 July 1895, 17, cited in Seraile, "Susan McKinney Steward," 31.

71. "Our Women Physicians," *Brooklyn Daily Times*, 27 June 1891, cited in Seraile, "Susan McKinney Steward," 33.

72. Seraile, "Susan McKinney Steward," 3, 39.

73. Susan McKinney Steward, "Women in Medicine," 17–18, as cited in Seraile, 39.

74. See, for example, Cott, *The Grounding of Modern Feminism*, 16–20; Jack S. Blocker

Jr., "Separate Paths: Suffragists and the Women's Temperance Crusade," *Signs* 10, no. 3 (spring 1985): 460–476; and Ellen Carol DuBois, *Feminism and Suffrage* (Ithaca, N.Y.: Cornell University Press, 1978).
75. Moldow, *Women Doctors in Gilded-Age Washington*, 142.
76. Rogers, "American Homeopathy Confronts Scientific Medicine," 38.
77. In February 1882, Members of the Medical Society of the State of New York adopted a "new code" allowing physicians to consult with any "legally qualified practitioners of medicine," violating the AMA's 1847 code prohibiting such interaction. The "old code" vs. new code" controversy was resolved in 1903 when the AMA replaced the old code with an advisory document liberalizing relations. See Kaufman, *Homeopathy in America*, 125–140, 154.
78. Erica Hearth of Brandeis University is writing a history of the WEIU and has generously provided me with a list of WEIU physicians between 1878–1924.
79. Moldow, *Women Doctors in Gilded-Age Washington*, 139.
80. Ibid., 147. See also Estelle Freedman, "Separatism as Strategy: Female Institution Building and American Feminism, 1870–1930," *Feminist Studies* 5, no. 3 (fall 1979): 512–529.
81. Ransom was vice president of the Professional Women's Club in 1907. Like other such organizations, members included both homeopathic and regular women physicians. For example, the committee in charge of the club's costume bazaar consisted of six homeopathic practitioners and ten regular physicians. Eliza Taylor Ransom Papers, 1888–1955, Schlesinger Library.
82. "At the Medical School," n.d., *Scrapbook*, Eliza Taylor Ransom papers.
83. Seraile, "Susan McKinney Steward," 40.
84. Sarah J. Millsop, M.D., "The South as a Field for Homeopaths," *Southern Journal of Homeopathy* 11 (November 1888): 383–384.
85. S. Penfield *New York Medical College and Hospital for Women Alumni Association Minutes, 1879*, 25, New York Academy of Medicine.
86. "Dr. Harriet French Dies of Paralysis," *Bradford Scrapbook*, vol. 5, 12. Sources differ on where in Philadelphia French received her medical training. An obituary in *Bradford Scrapbook* 5.12 notes she graduated from Hahnemann College, date unknown. However, since Hahnemann did not matriculate women, French may have attended informally without receiving an M.D. diploma. Another source indicates she graduated from the eclectic Penn Medical University, date unknown.
87. Ruth Thompson, "Minnesota Memories," *Minneapolis Tribune* 5 January 1948, n.p., Martha George Ripley Papers, 1880–1912.
88. For example, see Anna Manning Comfort, "Struggles and Trials of the Pioneer Medical Woman," *The Guilder* (May 1903): 17–24. *The Guilder* was a publication of the Hospital Guild of the NYMCHW.
89. "An Experienced Physician," *Syracuse Post*, 2 November 1896.
90. *Syracuse Herald*, Sunday, 6 October 1895.
91. Anna Howard Shaw, *The Story of a Pioneer* (New York and London: Harper & Brothers, 1915), 141.
92. BU's medical school identified itself as homeopathic until 1918.

Chapter 3 Becoming Physicians

1. Frances Janney Derby to Rebecca Smith Janney, 7 August 1874, Janney Family Papers, MSS 142, Ohio Historical Society.
2. Ibid.
3. Women's regular schools included Woman's Medical College of Pennsylvania, Philadelphia (1850); Women's Medical College of the New York Infirmary for

Women and Children, New York (1868); New England Female Medical College, Boston (1848); and Women's Hospital Medical College, Chicago (1870). From Mary Roth Walsh, *"Doctors Wanted No Women Need Apply," Sexual Barriers in the Medical Profession, 1835–1975* (New Haven: Yale University Press, 1977), 180.

4. The total increased from 272 graduates during the 1870s to 542 graduates during the 1880s. Numbers from Winston Database.

5. This college underwent several name changes over the years. Incorporated as the Western College of Homoeopathic Medicine in 1850, it became the Western College of Homoeopathy around 1859, the Western Homoeopathic Medical College in 1860–1861; and by 1870, the Cleveland Homoeopathic College.

6. Central Medical College of New York (eclectic) graduated Lydia Folger Fowler in 1850; Clemence Lozier graduated from its successor, the Syracuse Eclectic Medical College in 1853. In Worcester, Massachusetts, Lucinda Susannah Hall graduated in 1852 from another eclectic school. The eclectic Penn Medical University in Philadelphia was open to women from its inception in 1853. See Bertha Eugenia Loveland Selmon, "Early Development of Medical Opportunity for Women in the United States, 1850–1879," *Medical Woman's Journal* (January 1947).

7. According to the 1867 schedule, lectures averaged five per day, were one hour long, and continued from November through February.

8. William Harvey King, ed., *History of Homoeopathy and Its Institutions in America* 3 (New York and Chicago: Lewis Publishing Co., 1905), 13–28.

9. *Minutes of the Faculty*, Western College of Homoeopathy, 5 October 1867, Dittrick Museum of Medical History Archives, Cleveland, Ohio.

10. A. P. Ketchum and M. A. Ferris to "The Faculty the Western College of Homoeopathy," 11 November 1867, Dittrick Archives.

11. For a concise biography of Myra King Merrick, see Charlotte S. Newman, "Cleveland's First Woman Physician: Myra Merrick Struggled to Bring Medical Care to the Poor," in *The Gamut* 216 (spring 1989): 15–29.

12. See William Barlow and David O. Powell, "Homeopathy and Sexual Equality: The Controversy over Coeducation at Cincinnati's Pulte Medical College, 1873–1879," in *Women and Health in America: Historical Readings*, ed. Judith Walzer Leavitt (Madison: University of Wisconsin Press, 1984), 422–427.

13. *Minutes of the Faculty*, Western College of Homoeopathy, 25 May 1968.

14. D. H. Beckwith, *History of the Cleveland Homoeopathic College from 1850 to 1880* (Cleveland, Ohio: 1908), 40. Coeducation at most medical colleges at this time consisted of equal but separate education of the sexes in all or some laboratories and lectures.

15. Although three female-only homeopathic schools were founded in the nineteenth century, two closed after one session. Homeopaths in Saint Louis, Missouri, founded women's colleges on two occasions: Dix Homoeopathic Medical College of Missouri for the Education of Women was organized in 1868, and the Women's Medical College of Saint Louis was founded in 1883. See Thomas L. Bradford, *Homoeopathic Bibliography of the United States* (1892).

16. *Annual Announcement of the NYMCW, 1869.*

17. *Transactions of the Homoeopathic Medical Society of the State of New York* 12 (1876–1877).

18. Leonard Paul Wershub, *One Hundred Years of Medical Progress: A History of the New York Medical College Flower and Fifth Avenue Hospitals* (Springfield, Ill.: Charles C. Thomas, 1967), 150–153.

19. Regina Markell Morantz-Sanchez, *Sympathy and Science: Women Physicians in American Medicine* (New York: Oxford University Press, 1985), 73. Harvard instituted similar requirements in 1871, and the University of Pennsylvania followed in 1877.

20. For an analysis of requirements at regular women's schools, see Regina Morantz-Sanchez, *Sympathy and Science*, 64–89.

21. William G. Rothstein, *American Medical Schools and the Practice of Medicine* (New York: Oxford University Press, 1987), 53.

22. *Annual Announcement NYMCW, 1869,* 10. According to Morantz-Sanchez, New York students were particularly hostile to women, whereas in Boston and Chicago women were accepted quietly and without fanfare. See Morantz-Sanchez, *Sympathy and Science*, 164.

23. A. W. Lozier, "'In Memoriam' Clemence Sophia Lozier, M.D.," address given to the New York City Suffrage League, 1 November 1888, Verticle files, Archives and Special Collection on Women in Medicine and Homeopathy, Drexel University College of Medicine, Philadelphia.

24. Elizabeth Cady Stanton, "Tribute to Dr. Clemence S. Lozier" delivered before the Woman's League, New York City, (7 June 1888), 40–41, Women Physicians Collection, ASCWMH.

25. King, ed., *History of Homoeopathy* 3 (1905), 133, 135, 154.

26. Lozier, "In Memoriam," 14.

27. King, ed., *History of Homoeopathy* 3 (1905), 154–155.

28. Phoebe J. Wait, Extracts from address at the opening exercises of New York Medical College and Hospital for Women, 1 October 1888, 35, Women Physicians Collection, ASCWMH.

29. Wershub, *One Hundred Years of Medical Progress*, 153.

30. *Annual Announcement of the NYMCW, 1893–1894, 1908–1909;* and *Cressett* 1, no. 5 (March 1898): 63.

31. *The Revolution*, 2, no. 9 (9 July 1868). Anthony patronized at least two women homeopaths: Julia Holmes Smith of Chicago and Marcena Sherman Ricker. Ricker, a gynecologist on the staff of the elite Rochester Homoeopathic Hospital, Rochester, N.Y. in 1906, also founded the Baptist Home in nearby Fairport and Door of Hope Home in Rochester. In 1931 she was an international delegate for the WCTU.

32. Bertha L. Selmon, "The New York Medical College and Hospital for Women" (April 1946), 43.

33. Anna Manning Comfort, "Women In Medicine (Then and Now)," Comfort Family Papers.

34. For a concise examination of the lives and experiences of African American women physicians in the nineteenth and early-twentieth centuries, see Darlene Clark Hine, "Co-Laborers in the Work of the Lord," in *The Racial Economy of Science: Toward a Democratic Future*, ed. Sandra Harding (Bloomington, Ind.: Indiana University Press, 1993). Also see Dorothy Sterling, ed., *We Are Your Sisters: Black Women in the Nineteenth Century* (New York: W. W. Norton & Co., 1984), 441–443.

35. William Seraile, "Susan McKinney Steward: New York State's First African American Woman Physician," *Afro-Americans in New York Life and History* 9, no. 2 (1985), 27–44.

36. Barlow and Powell, "Homeopathy and Sexual Equality," 422–428.

37. Clarke published *Sex in Education; or, A Fair Chance for Girls* in 1873, and while not all physicians accepted his theories, *Sex in Education* underwent seventeen revisions during the next thirteen years and provoked wide debate. See Vern Bullough and Martha Voght, "Women, Menstruation, and Nineteenth-Century Medicine," in *Bulletin of the History of Medicine* 47 (1973): 66–82.

38. Tullio Suzzara Verdi, M.D., *Mothers and Daughters: Practical Studies for the Conservation of the Health of Girls* (1877), 201–202.

39. Frank F. Laird, "Gynaecology vs. Coeducation" (M.D. thesis, Hahnemann Medical College of Philadelphia, 1880).

40. See Regina Markell Morantz, "The 'Connecting Link': The Case for the Woman Doctor in Nineteenth Century America," in *Sickness and Health in America: Readings in the History of Medicine and Public Health*, ed. Judith Walzer Leavitt and Ronald L. Numbers, rev. 2d ed., (Madison: University of Wisconsin Press, 1985), 161–172.

41. Nine schools admitting women include: state universities in Michigan and Iowa, where women were admitted to regular and homeopathic medical departments; Homoeopathic Medical College of Missouri; Chicago Homoeopathic College; Boston University School of Medicine; Western College of Homoeopathy in Cleveland; the New York Medical College and Hospital for Women; Pulte Medical College, Cincinnati; and Hahnemann Medical College of Chicago.

42. A. R. Thomas to Drs. Sartain, et. al. of the Women's Medical Club of Philadelphia, September 1884, Sartain Collection, Historical Society of Pennsylvania.

43. See Naomi Rogers, *An Alternative Path: The Making and Remaking of Hahnemann Medical College and Hospital of Philadelphia* (New Brunswick, N.J.: Rutgers University Press, 1998).

44. "A. R. Thomas to Drs. Sartain, et. al.," 1 September 1886, in *An Alternative Path: The Making and Remaking of Hahnemann Medical College and Hospital of Philadelphia* (New Brunswick, N.J.: Rutgers University Press, 1998).

45. King, ed., *History of Homoeopathy* 2 (1905), 345–350.

46. *First Annual Report of the Massachusetts Homoeopathic Hospital and the Ladies' Aid Association*, 10 September 1871; and *Annual Report*, September 1877. The Ladies' Aid Association acquired 348 members within its first year of organization.

47. King, ed., *History of Homoeopathy* 3 (1905), 180–181, 187–88.

48. Walsh, *"Doctors Wanted: No Women Need Apply,"* 71.

49. King, ed., *History of Homoeopathy* 3 (1905), 186.

50. For a discussion of education reforms during this period, see Kenneth M. Ludmerer, *Learning to Heal: The Development of American Medical Education* (New York: Basic Books, 1985), 72–101.

51. Earl H. Dearborn, "The Development of Pharmacology at Boston University School of Medicine," *The Boston Medical Quarterly* 6, no. 2 (June 1955): 34. As Ted J. Kaptchuk notes, homeopaths were the first group to routinely adopt blind assessment in their evaluation of homeopathic remedies. See "Intentional Ignorance: A History of Blind Assessment and Placebo Controls in Medicine," *Bulletin of the History of Medicine* 72 (1998): 389–433.

52. Morantz-Sanchez, *Sympathy and Science*, 122–123.

53. Frances Janney Derby to Rebecca Smith Janney and Anne Janney Deming, 7 October 1874, Janney Family Papers, MSS 142, Ohio Historical Society.

54. Frances Janney Derby to Anne Janney Deming, 18 October 1874, Janney Papers.

55. Frances Janney Derby to Janney Family, 20 December 1874, Janney Papers.

56. Frances Janney Derby to Rebecca Smith Janney, 21 October 1875, Janney Papers.

57. Ibid., 16 January (no year).

58. Frances Janney Derby to John Jay Janney and Rebecca Smith Janney, 12 December 1875, Janney Papers.

59. Ibid., 13 February 1876.

60. Frances Janney Derby to Rebecca Smith Janney, 30 December 1876, Janney Papers.

61. Frances Janney Derby to Anne Janney Deming, 17 December no year, Janney Papers.

62. Frances Janney Derby to Janney Family, 18 February no year, Janney Papers.
63. Frances Janney Derby to Anne Janney Deming, 14 January 1877, Janney Papers.
64. Frances Janney Derby to Rebecca Smith Janney, 15 January 1877, Janney Papers.
65. Frances Janney Derby to John Jay Janney, no date, Janney Papers.
66. Frances Janney Derby to Rebecca Smith Janney, 7 August 1874, Janney Papers.
67. Frances Janney Derby to Anne Janney Deming, 12 November 1876, Janney Papers.
68. Ibid.
69. Thomas Neville Bonner, *To the Ends of the Earth: Women's Search for Education in Medicine* (Cambridge: Harvard University Press, 1992), 140. The homeopathic medical department at the State University of Michigan in Ann Arbor was not instituted until 1875.
70. Morantz-Sanchez, *Sympathy and Science*, 113.
71. Frances Janney Derby to Anne Janney Deming, 21 November 1876, Janney Papers. Ohio Historical Society.
72. Frances Janney Derby to Janney Family, 18 January 1875, Janney Papers.
73. Frances Janney Derby to Rebecca Smith Janney and John Jay Janney, 3 April 1875, Janney Papers.
74. Frances Janney Derby to Anne Janney Deming, 18 October 1874, Janney Papers.
75. Frances Janney Derby to Janney Family, 20 December 1874, Janney Papers.
76. Frances Janney Derby to Rebecca Smith Janney, 31 January 1875, Janney Papers.
77. Ibid., 23 May 1875.
78. Ibid., 16 January (no year).
79. Ibid., 9 June 1875.
80. Ibid., 23 May 1875.
81. Morantz-Sanchez, *Sympathy and Science*, 73.
82. Frances Janney Derby to Anne Janney Deming, 14 May (no year), Janney Papers.
83. Mary Safford Blake, "Boston News," *The Medical Investigator* 11, no. 121 (January 1874): 250.
84. Naomi Rogers, "Women and Sectarian Medicine," in *Women, Health, and Medicine in America: A Historical Handbook*, ed. Rima D. Apple (New Brunswick, N.J.: Rutgers University Press, 1990), 290.
85. "Graduates of Homoeopathic Medical Colleges. Session of 1898–1899," in *Transactions of the AIH* (1899): 775–776.
86. According to Ellen More, Sarah Adamson Dolly, an 1852 graduate of the eclectic Central Medical College, claimed she had no idea distinctions between "regular" and "irregular" medical schools even existed. See Ellen Singer More, *Restoring the Balance: Women Physicians and the Profession of Medicine, 1850–1995* (Cambridge: Harvard University Press, 1999), 21.
87. Dr. May D. Hanks, interview by Mary Ware Dennett, Chicago, 11 February 1927, National Center for Homeopathy Archives, Alexandria, Va.
88. *Transactions of the Alumnae Association of WMCP, 1896:* 73–74. I assume this phrase, the "practice of warming a viper," refers to unorthodox practice in general, but am unsure of its precise meaning.
89. Dr. S. Mary Ives, "Obituary," Woman Physicians Collection, ASCWMH.
90. Lydia Webster Stokes, Woman Physicians Collection. Members of the Alumnae Association of WMCP relaxed their vigilance against associating with unorthodox colleagues when they invited "our Homeopathic alumnae" to join the organization in January 1914. See *Transactions of the Alumnae Association, WMCP, January 1914:* 34.
91. Of the thirty women I have identified as "converts," graduation dates are known

for twenty-six. While fifteen women graduated from regular schools between 1890 and 1899, the remaining eleven graduated within a thirty-year period beginning in 1859.

Chapter 4 Adding Women to the Ranks

1. "The Admission of Women," *Transactions of the American Institute of Homoeopathy*, 1869–1870: 345.
2. Amelia J. Burroughs, M.D., "Women in the American Institute of Homoeopathy," *Medical Century* 11, no. 13 (1894): 314.
3. Several scholars discuss the function of medical societies and their relationship to medical licensing, including William G. Rothstein, *American Physicians in the Nineteenth Century: From Sects to Science* (Baltimore: Johns Hopkins University Press, 1985), 63–121; Joseph F. Kett, *The Formation of the American Medical Profession: The Role of Institutions, 1780–1860* (New Haven: Yale University Press, 1968).
4. For studies on women's admission to medical societies, see Martin Kaufman, "The Admission of Women to Nineteenth-Century American Medical Societies," *Bulletin of the History of Medicine* 50 (1976): 251–260; Ellen More, "The Blackwell Medical Society and the Professionalization of Women Physicians," *Bulletin of the History of Medicine* 61 (1987): 603–628; Phoebe Peck, "Women Physicians and Their State Medical Societies," *Journal of the American Medicine Women's Association* 20, no. 4 (1965): 351–353; and Cora Bagley Marrett, "On the Evolution of Women's Medical Societies," *Bulletin of the History of Medicine* 53 (1979): 434–448.
5. On the sexual separatism of women in the regular medical profession, for example, see Virginia G. Drachman, "The Limits of Progress: The Professional Lives of Women Doctors, 1881–1926," *Bulletin of the History of Medicine* 60 (spring 1986): 56–72.
6. *Proceedings of the IHA* from 1896 to 1915.
7. *Transactions of the AIH* for various years.
8. See Appendix A for a more complete listing of women on committees and executive boards of homeopathic medical societies.
9. In 1899, the Homoeopathic Medical Society of the State of New York was the largest with 509 members; Pennsylvania was second with 318; and Illinois was third with 294 members. *Transactions of the AIH* (1899).
10. "Homoeopathy, Scientific Medicine, Excelsior," *The United States Medical Investigator* 17 (1882): 86–87.
11. *Medical Century* 3, no. 14 (1895): 335; and *Transactions of the AIH* (1895): 146.
12. Reference is to medical societies that were not restricted to alumnae of educational institutions.
13. Marrett, "On the Evolution of Women's Medical Societies," in *Women and Health in America*, ed. Judith Walzer Leavitt (Madison: University of Wisconsin Press, 1984), 433.
14. *Journal of the American Institute of Homoeopathy* 18, no. 1 (January 1925): 84.
15. One source indicates that Sartain retired in 1889, which means that the women's medical club was in existence for at least part of the 1890s. From "Harriet Judd Sartain, M.D.," Sartain Collection, box 7, Historical Society of Pennsylvania.
16. More, "The Blackwell Medical Society and the Professionalization of Women Physicians," 604. Also see Estelle Freedman, "Separatism as Strategy: Female Institution Building and American Feminism," *Feminist Studies* 53 (1979): 512–529; Cora Bagley Marrett, "Influences on the Rise of New Organizations: The Forma-

tion of Women's Medical Societies," *Administrative Science Quarterly* 25 (June 1980): 432, 439; and Regina Morantz-Sanchez, *Sympathy and Science: Women Physicians in American Medicine* (New York: Oxford University Press, 1985), 180–181.

17. Morantz-Sanchez, *Sympathy and Science*, 180.

18. Figures are from various issues of state medical society proceedings.

19. Because of their smaller numbers, homeopaths organized few independent specialty societies. In their place were specialty sections or "bureaus" within national and state societies. According to Rothstein, these intraorganizational sections developed more rapidly within the AIH than in the AMA. See *American Physicians in the Nineteenth Century*, 236.

20. *Transactions of the Homoeopathic Medical Society of the State of Pennsylvania* (1881–1900).

21. *Transactions of the Medical Society of Pennsylvania* (1882–1900).

22. Percentages compiled from physicians listed in *The Physicians' and Dentists' Directory of the States of Pennsylvania, New Jersey, and Delaware* (Philadelphia: P. F. Young & Co.). Although no date appears on the directory, the numbers of women in practice in Philadelphia around 1897 correspond to listings in R. L. Polk, ed., *Medical and Surgical Register of the United States and Canada* (1896–1898).

23. Morantz-Sanchez, *Sympathy and Science*, 182–183.

24. Not all women, of course, rejected the new ideas of science and professionalism. Like Mary Putnam Jacobi and Mary Dixon Jones, those who found them compatible with their own ideas of women's role in the profession tended to be very active in a variety of medical societies. For example, see Regina Morantz-Sanchez, "Entering Male Professional Terrain: Dr. Mary Dixon Jones and the Emergence of Gynecological Surgery in the Nineteenth-Century United States," *Gender and History* 7, no. 2 (August 1995): 201–221.

25. More, "Blackwell Medical Society," 607; and *Restoring the Balance: Women Physicians and the Profession of Medicine, 1850–1995* (Cambridge: Harvard University Press, 1999), 42–69.

26. Morantz-Sanchez, *Sympathy and Science*, 70; and "The Gendering of Empathic Expertise: How Women Physicians Became More Empathic than Men," in *The Empathic Practitioner: Empathy, Gender, and Medicine*, ed. Ellen Singer More and Maureen A. Milligan, (New Bunswick, N.J.: Rutgers University Press, 1994), 40–58. Also see Ellen Singer More, "'Empathy' Enters the Profession of Medicine," in *The Empathic Practitioner*, 19–39.

27. Ruben Ludlam, "Annual Address", 346; "The Admission of Women," *Transactions of the AIH* (1869): 61; and Ludlam, "Woman and Homoeopathy," *Transactions of the AIH* (1869): 367.

28. Carroll Dunham, "Liberty of Medical Opinion and Action: A Vital Necessity and a Great Responsibility" (annual address delivered before the AIH, 8 June 1870); reprint, *Transactions of the Homoeopathic Medical Society of the State of New York* 8 (1870): 742.

29. Carroll Dunham, "Lilium-Tigrinum—A Summary of a Few Provings Upon Women," *North American Journal of Homoeopathy* 1, no. 11 (November 1870): 160.

30. David Thayer, "Annual Address," Proceedings of the Annual Meeting, 1870, *Publications of the Massachusetts Homoeopathic Medical Society, 1866–1870*, (1875), 526–527.

31. Roberts Bartholow, "Cui Bono? And What Nature, What Art Does in the Cure of Disease" (two introductory lectures delivered in the Medical College of Ohio, 1872–1873 and 1873–1874, Cincinnati: Clarke, 1873), 17, in John Harley

Warner, *The Therapeutic Perspective: Medical Practice, Knowledge, and Identity in America, 1820–1885* (Cambridge: Harvard University Press, 1986), 263–264.

32. J. Henry Allen, "President's Address," *Proceedings of the IHA* (1900): 1–5; also see Harris L. Coulter, *Divided Legacy: The Conflict between Homoeopathy and the American Medical Association*, 2d ed. (Richmond, Calif.: North Atlantic Books, 1982), 328–370.

33. C. Pearson, "History of the Society," *Proceedings of the IHA* (1881–1883): 5.

34. W. E. Payne, "Miscellaneous Items," *North American Journal of Homoeopathy* (1871), n.s.: 1 (3), 430.

35. "The Admission of Women," (1869), 346.

36. "Original Communications," *The Richmond and Louisville Medical Journal* 12, no. 1 (July 1871): 27, 17.

37. Morantz-Sanchez, *Sympathy and Science*, 179; and Ellen S. More, "The American Medical Women's Association and the Role of the Woman Physician, 1915–1990," *Journal of the American Medical Women's Association* 45, no. 5 (September/October 1990): 165.

38. *Transactions of the Homoeopathic Medical Society of the State of Pennsylvania* (1872).

39. Emily Sartain to Frank Weitenkampf, 10 April 1888, in Phyllis Peet, "The Emergence of American Women Printmakers in the Late Nineteenth Century," (Ph.D. diss., University of California at Los Angeles, 1987), 615.

40. Harriet Judd Sartain, M.D., Sartain Collection, box 7, Historical Society of Pennsylvania.

41. Pemberton Dudley, M.D., ed., *Directory of the Homoeopathic Physicians of the State of Pennsylvania* (1874). The number of women homeopaths represents approximately 6 percent of all homeopaths in the city. While privately published medical directories are subject to great inaccuracies, at times they provide the only ballpark figures to be had. Census records do not distinguish sectarian from regular practitioners, and city directories of this period often do not identify physicians as a separate category from residents.

42. See Kaufman, "The Admission of Women to Nineteenth-Century American Medical Societies," 251–260; and *Homeopathy in America*, 54–55.

43. Penn Medical University graduated ninety-three women physicians by 1879. See Harold J. Abrahams, *Extinct Medical Schools of Nineteenth-Century Philadelphia* (Philadelphia: University of Pennsylvania Press, 1966), 176–231.

44. Whitfield J. Bell Jr., *The College of Physicians of Philadelphia: A Bicentennial History* (Philadelphia: Science History Publications, 1987), 143; and Ellen Singer More, "The Professionalism of Sarah Dolley, M.D.," in *Restoring the Balance: Women Physicians and the Profession of Medicine, 1850–1995* (Cambridge: Harvard University Press, 1999), 13–41.

45. "The Recognition of Female Physicians by the Medical Profession of Pennsylvania," *A Brief History of Proceedings in the Medical Society of Pennsylvania in the Years 1859, 1860, 1867, 1868, 1870, and 1871 to Procure the Recognition of Women Physicians* (1894), 10–24.

46. "Original Communications," 23–24, 33.

47. Fellows of the College did not disrupt the harmony or esprit de corps of their own institution by admitting women until 1932. See Bell Jr., *The College of Physicians of Philadelphia*, 251–252. For a discussion of the stratification and specialization of medical societies, see Rothstein, *American Physicians in the Nineteenth Century*, 198–216.

48. "Original Communications," 54–55.

49. According to 1870 Census statistics, Philadelphia had 1,077 physicians in a population of 674,022. New York City's population was 942,292 with 1,741 physicians.

Statistics from the Ninth Census of the United States, 1870, vol. 2, (1872), 794, 254, 212, 793.

50. Bell, *The College of Physicians of Philadelphia*, 142–145.
51. Of the twenty-six, nine were homeopaths and seventeen were regulars according to ed., Samuel W. Butler, *The Medical Register and Directory of the U.S.*, (1874). With a city population of 674,022, physicians practicing in Philadelphia (regular and irregular) totaled 1,205.
52. These numbers are approximate and are based on physicians listed in Butler.
53. "The Recognition of Female Physicians by the Medical Profession of Pennsylvania," *A Brief History*, 10–24.
54. Peck, "Women Physicians and their State Medical Societies," 353.
55. *Transactions of the Medical Society of Pennsylvania* (1882–1900).
56. Bell Jr., *The College of Physicians of Philadelphia*, 145.
57. Mary Roth Walsh, *"Doctors Wanted: No Women Need Apply" Sexual Barriers in the Medical Profession, 1835–1975* (New Haven: Yale University Press, 1977), 150–151.
58. William Harvey King, ed., *History of Homoeopathy*, vol. 3, (1905), 172.
59. Samuel Augustus Fisk, A.L.S. to Dr. William Williamson Wellington, Northampton, Mass., 26 September 1875, Francis A. Countway Library of Medicine, B MS/c75.2, 3–4, Harvard University.
60. *Boston City Directory, 1870*. Introduced by Charles Baunscheidt in Germany about 1860, Baunscheidtism was a counter-irritation therapy, in which a disc-like instrument with a ring of needles applied to the skin was thought to divert the nervous activity from the inner organs to the surface of the body, creating external warmth and relieving congestions and inflammations. See John Linden *Manual of the Exanthematic Method of Cure, Also Known as Baunscheidtism* (Cleveland, 1903).
61. See Thomas Neville Bonner, *To the Ends of the Earth: Women's Search for Education in Medicine* (Cambridge: Harvard University Press, 1992).
62. "Minority Report," 6 October 1875, Francis A. Countway Library of Medicine, B MS/c75.2, Harvard University.
63. According to Polk's *Directory*, there were seventeen women regulars and twenty-seven women homeopaths. However, fifty-three women lacked any designation. From the *Medical and Surgical Directory of the United States*, ed. R. L. Polk (1886).
64. Henry Ingersoll Bowditch, "Majority Report on Accepting Women into the Massachusetts Medical Society," 1 October 1875, Countway Library of Medicine, B MX/c75.2.
65. From the records of the Massachusetts Medical Society and the Chadwick Scrapbook cited in Walsh, *"Doctors Wanted: No Women Need Apply,"* 160–161.

Chapter 5   *"Women's Diseases" and Homeopathic Patients*

1. T. G. Comstock, M.D., "Flexions of the Uterus," *Transactions of the AIH, 1869* (1870): 298–305.
2. Ibid., 302. Sounds were long, pointed tools of various lengths. Insertion into the cervix and uterus was meant to relieve menstrual irregularities caused by constriction or "congestion" and to reposition the uterus in cases of displacements. Uterine "displacements" variously referred to prolapse or falling of the womb; backward displacements, including retroversions and retroflexions; and the forward displacements of anteversions and anteflexions.
3. Ibid., 303–304.
4. Charles E. Rosenberg, "The Therapeutic Revolution: Medicine, Meaning, and Social Change in Nineteenth-Century America," ed. Judith Walzer Leavitt and

Ronald L. Numbers, *Sickness and Health in America: Readings in the History of Medicine and Public Health* (Madison: University of Wisconsin Press, 1985), 41.

5. Harris L. Coulter, *Divided Legacy: The Conflict Between Homoeopathy and the American Medical Association, Science and Ethics in American Medicine, 1800–1914,* 2d ed. (Berkeley, Calif.: North Atlantic Books, 1982), 114.

6. Regina Morantz-Sanchez, *Sympathy and Science: Women Physicians in American Medicine* (New York: Oxford University Press, 1985), 56.

7. W. B. Clarke, "Homoeopathy in Obstetrics" (M.D. thesis, Homoeopathic Medical College of Pennsylvania, 1852).

8. Thomas Skinner, M.D., *Homoeopathy in its Relation to the Diseases of Women* (1876), 31–35.

9. Fistulas are openings or holes created between the vagina and neighboring organs. Vesicovaginal fistulas (between bladder and vagina) and rectovaginal (between the rectum and vagina) occurred when the infant's head rested for long periods in the vagina, cutting off circulation to surrounding tissues. Fistulas were often created when forceps or a perforation hook was used as aids to end labor. See Edward Shorter, *Women's Bodies: A Social History of Women's Encounter with Health, Ill-Health, and Medicine* (New Brunswick, N.J.: Transaction Publishers, 1991), 268–275.

10. Obadiah G. Brickley, "The Uterus and its Appendages" (M.D. thesis, Hahnemann Medical College of Pennsylvania, 1855).

11. I would like to thank Lenette E. Leidy whose paper, "Social Roles and Uterine Position: Nineteenth-Century Therapeutics for Prolapse," presented at the 1995 session of the American Association of the History of Medicine, broadened my thinking on the social meanings of menstruation and uterine displacements.

12. Carroll Smith-Rosenberg and Charles E. Rosenberg, "The Female Animal: Medical and Biological Views of Woman and Her Role in Nineteenth-Century America," in *Women and Health in America: Historical Readings,* ed. Judith Walzer Leavitt (Madison: University of Wisconsin Press, 1984).

13. Sources include: Lawson Tait, *Diseases of Women* (1877), 145. Although Tait was a regular physician his text was used in homeopathic as well as regular medical colleges: D. C. Kline, "Advice to Girls at Puberty," CPP pamphlet *Gynecology* 245, 1–3; and Constantine Hering, *Domestic Physician,* 4th American rev. ed., (1848), 292–293. Alexandra Lord shows that eighteenth as well as nineteenth-century views of menstruation drew on models from ancient and medieval medicine. Although different in some respects, they did not differ radically from past theories. See Alexandra Lord, "'The Great *Arcana* of the Deity': Menstruation and Menstrual Disorders in Eighteenth-Century British Medical Thought," *Bulletin of the History of Medicine* 73, no.1 (spring 1999): 38–63.

14. Walter Williamson, "Diseases of Females and Children," in Constantine Hering's *Domestic Physician* (1848), 295–296.

15. E. D. Paine, "Cases of Practice," *The Homoeopathic Examiner* 3 (1844).

16. "A Few Words on the Use of Cold Water Injections in Uterine Hemorrhage," in *The Homoeopathic Examiner* 9 (April 1847): 386–387.

17. Williamson, "Diseases of Females and Children," 311. Pessaries were designed for several purposes but primarily to retain a dislocated uterus. Made from a variety of materials including glass, silver, brass, wood, ivory, bone, wax, cork, leather, and sponge, some were constructed to maintain the vagina in a position of constant dilation, while others were in the shape of a stem protruding from a cup or ball. Pessaries constructed of porus materials sometimes were impregnated with acetate of lead and opium for local applications of drugs. See Tait, *Diseases of Women* (1877). Over four hundred different types had been devised for use by European

and American women and were either procured from one's practitioner, ordered by mail, or fashioned by the woman herself.

18. *Transactions of the Alumnae Association of the Woman's Medical College of Pennsylvania* (1884): 27–28.

19. Henry N. Guernsey, M.D., *Guernsey's Obstetrics. The Application of the Principles and Practice of Homoeopathy to Obstetrics and the Disorders Peculiar to Women and Young Children*, 3rd ed. (1886), 631–632.

20. Henry N. Guernsey, M.D., "Report on Obstetrics," *Transactions of the AIH* (1869): 328.

21. Ibid., 329–333.

22. At a later date, Dr. Guernsey claimed that in his thirty-five year practice, having treated four thousand cases of childbed sickness, "I have, *truthfully* and *honestly*, never lost a case by uterine haemorrhage, and I have *never* used an adjuvant of any sort or kind." See "A Treatise by Henry N. Guernsey, M.D.," read before the New York County Homoeopathic Medical Society, 13 November 1878; reprint, *New York Homoeopathic Times* (January 1879), CPP pamphlet, *Obstetrics/Gynaecology* 159.

23. Samuel Hahnemann, *Organon*, 5th and 6th eds., 103–104.

24. From the standpoint of physicians, pessaries, intrauterine douches, and sponges supposedly corrected cervical and uterine irregularities, conditions which interfered with women's ability to conceive and bear children. But women's acceptance and even demands for these devices indicate another use. As Linda Gordon argues, there was never any doubt that they were used as birth control devices. Pessaries and suppositories were usually able to be removed and replaced by women themselves and appeared to be in great demand. See Linda Gordon, *Woman's Body, Woman's Right: Birth Control in America*, rev. ed. (New York: Penguin Books, 1990), 67–68.

25. Ruben Ludlam, M.D., "Notes on Mechanical Dysmenorrhoea," *North American Journal of Homoeopathy* 10, no. 37 (August 1861): 64.

26. Comstock, "Flexions of the Uterus," 302–303.

27. Called "white flower" epidemics among industrial workers, leukorrhea is a modern term for a variety of vaginal or uterine discharges. Physicians considered it a separate disease rather than symptom of other underlying causes. The prevalence of leukorrhoea among women in the textile and shoe industries during the second half of the nineteenth century caused physicians to conclude it was caused by long periods of sitting. See Edward Shorter, *The History of Women's Bodies* (New York: Basic Books, 1982), 255–263.

28. A. M. Cushing, M.D., "The Homoeopathic Treatment of Diseases Peculiar to Women," read before the Homoeopathic Medical Society of Western Massachusetts, 16 December 1898, CPP pamphlet, *Homoeopathy* 169, 3.

29. James Tyler Kent, M.D., "Ovarian Tumor with Lycopod," *Proceedings of International Hahnemannian Association*, 1892 (1893): 178.

30. T. M. Dinningham, M.D., "Homoeopathy and Gynecology," *Proceedings of the IHA* (1890): 172.

31. P. P. Wells, review of *Uterine Therapeutics*, by H. Minton, M.D., *The Homoeopathic Physician* 3 (3 March 1884): 75–76.

32. Anna Manning Comfort, *Record Book, 1867*, Comfort Family Papers.

33. Mrs. E. G. Cook, M.D., "On the Use of Intrauterine Stem Pessaries," *Transactions of the AIH* (1880): 466–473.

34. H. C. Clapp, M.D., "Ulceration of the Os Uteri," *New England Medical Gazette* 9, no. 7 (1874): 330.

35. J. C. Burgher, M.D., "Displacements of the Uterus," *Transactions of the AIH*

(1876): 520.

36. Naomi Rogers, An Alternative Path: The Making and Remaking of Hahnemann Medical College and Hospital of Philadelphia (New Brunswick, N.J.: Rutgers University Press, 1998), 27, 124.

37. Sarah J. Millsop, M.D., "Are Homoeopaths Good Diagnosticians?" Southern Journal of Homoeopathy 3, no. 9 (December 1890): 320.

38. Ibid., 319.

39. Mary A. Brinkman, M.D., "The Relation of Homoeopathy to Gynaecology; or Sectarianism in Medicine," Homoeopathic Journal of Obstetrics 12 (1890): 170.

40. James V. Ricci provides a richly detailed overview of gynecological procedures and technological developments in The Development of Gynaecological Surgery and Instruments: A Comprehensive Review of the Evolution of Surgery and Surgical Instruments for the Treatment of Female Diseases from the Hippocratic Age to the Antiseptic Period (Philadelphia and Toronto: The Blakiston Co., 1949). See also Christopher Lawrence, "Democratic, Divine, and Heroic: The History and Historiography of Surgery," in Medical Theory, Surgical Practice: Studies in the History of Surgery, ed. Lawrence (London: Routledge, 1992); and Regina Morantz-Sanchez, Conduct Unbecoming a Woman: Medicine on Trial in Turn-of-the-Century Brooklyn (New York: Oxford University Press, 1999), 88–113.

41. William Todd Helmuth, "Surgery in the Homeopathic School," Medical Century 1, no. 6 (June 1893): 192–197.

42. James Tyler Kent, Lectures on Homoeopathic Philosophy (1900; reprint, Berkeley, Calif.: North Atlantic Books, 1979), 47–48.

43. Sarah J. Millsop, "Diseases of Women Cured Without the Knife," Transactions of the AIH (1895): 469.

44. William G. Rothstein, American Physicians in the Nineteenth Century, 259.

45. The National Cyclopaedia of American Biography 7 (1897), 269–270.

46. Biographical material on William Todd Helmuth is from History of Homoeopathy and Its Institutions in America, ed. William Harvey King (New York: Lewis Publishing Co., 1905), 4: 69–70. For surgical statistics and information on Helmuth House see: The Hahnemannian Monthly 10 (October 1887): 594–602. As Paul Starr notes, many physicians established small private hospitals in order to accommodate patients' desires for privacy and to counter their fears of hospitalization by providing nursing and hotel services. See The Social Transformation of American Medicine (New York: Basic Books, 1982), 157.

47. Twenty-eighth Annual Report of the Massachusetts Homoeopathic Hospital and Alumni Association, 31 December 1897, 28–29.

48. Surgical and medical data collected from individual case records of patients admitted to the Massachusetts Homoeopathic Hospital during the month of July 1897 and between November 1–21, 1897.

49. For a useful historiography of surgical gynecology see Judith M. Roy, "Surgical Gynecology," in Women, Health, and Medicine in America: A Historical Handbook, ed. Rima D. Apple (New Brunswick, N.J.: Rutgers University Press, 1990), 173–195.

50. Millsop, "Diseases of Women Cured Without the Knife," Transactions of the AIH (1895): 469.

51. Regina Morantz-Sanchez explores the career strategies of Dr. Mary Dixon Jones, noting the permeability of boundaries between specialty areas and general practice that existed well into the first decade of the twentieth century. See "Entering Male Professional Terrain: Dr. Mary Dixon Jones and the Emergence of Gynecological Surgery in the Nineteenth-Century United States," Gender and History 7, no. 2 (August 1995): 201–221. Specialization in the nineteenth century meant that a

physician's interest and medical practice centered on a particular area of medicine. Declaring a specialty required no formal examinations or membership in organizations until the twentieth century. See Charles E. Rosenberg, ed., *The Origins of Specialization in American Medicine: An Anthology of Sources* (New York and London: Garland Publishing, 1989); and Rosemary Stevens, "The Changing Idea of a Medical Specialty," *Transactions and Studies of the College of Physicians of Philadelphia* 5 (1980): 159–177.

52. *Transactions of the AIH* (1894): 637.
53. Dewitt G. Wilcox, M.D., "Obstetric Surgery," CPP pamphlet, *Gynecology* 245, 1–2.
54. Sarah J. Lee, M.D., "Can Laceration of the Perineum Be Prevented?" *Homoeopathic Journal of Obstetrics* 11, no. 1 (January 1889): 136.
55. *Transactions of the AIH* (1880): 478.
56. "Report of the Section in Obstetrics," *Transactions of the AIH* (1894).
57. Women doctors often paid greater attention to preventive medicine, emphasizing patient education and milder therapies—including placebos—before turning to stronger drugs or more invasive procedures. See Morantz-Sanchez, *Sympathy and Science*, 214–216.
58. "Report," *Transactions of the AIH* (1894): 637.
59. Florence N. Ward, M.D., "Improved Technique for the Primary Repair of Lacerations of the Pelvic Floor," *Transactions of the AIH* (1903): 555.
60. Ibid., 565–566.
61. Lizzie Gray Gutherz, M.D., "Woman's Steadfast Friend," *Transactions of the AIH* (1894): 735–736.
62. S. P. Hedges, M.D., "Plea for a Return to the Use of Our Remedies in Gynecology," *Medical Century* 4, no. 11 (1 June 1896): 260–262.
63. Martin Pernick, *A Calculus of Suffering: Pain, Professionalism, and Anesthesia in Nineteenth-Century America* (New York: Columbia University Press, 1985), 101–102.
64. "Report on the Section in Gynaecology," *Transactions of the AIH* (1894): 789, 791.
65. See for example Ann Douglas Wood, "The Fashionable Diseases": Women's Complaints and Their Treatment in Nineteenth-Century America," in *Women and Health in America*, ed. Leavitt, 222–238. For a critique of Wood's presentist, polemical slant, see Regina Morantz-Sanchez, "The Perils of Feminist History," *Women and Health in America*, 239–245.
66. Dr. Theodore Gramm, "Two Cases of Caesarean Section," *The Hahnemannian Monthly* (August 1899; reprint, CPP pamphlet, *Obstetrics/Gynecology* 156), 6. The surgical procedure of craniotomy involved perforating the skull of the fetus, evacuating the brain, and reducing the size of the head in cases where it was disproportionately larger than the parturient canal. By 1890, physicians debated whether this procedure was ever justifiable given recent advances and improvements in the techniques of Caesarean section.
67. J. J. Thompson, M.D., "The Hysterectomy Fad," *Transactions of the AIH* (1895), 484; and J. Martin Kershaw, M.D., "Are the Nervous Manifestations of Pelvic Disease Removed by Castration?" *Southern Journal of Homoeopathy* (n.d.). For a discussion of women's demand for gynecological surgery, see Edward Shorter, *From Paralysis to Fatigue: A History of Psychosomatic Illness in the Modern Era* (New York: The Free Press, 1992), 86–94; and Morantz-Sanchez, *Conduct Unbecoming a Woman*, 106. For a discussion on the use of the terms "oophorectomy" and "ovariotomy," see *Conduct Unbecoming*, 96–101. The following authors show the influence of professional ambition and rivalry as well as public opinion on the popularity of Battey's operation: Lawrence D. Longo, "The Rise and Fall of Battey's

Operation: A Fashion in Surgery," *Bulletin of the History of Medicine* 53 (1979): 244–267; and Andrew Scull and Diane Favreau, "A Chance to Cut is a Chance to Cure," *Research in Law, Deviance, and Social Control* 8 (1986): 3–39.

68. Nancy Theriot argues that women were equally responsible with physicians for the dominance of the gynecological perspective. I believe she overstates the case. Women's ideas of illness were constructed within a theoretical framework developed and revised by male physicians since the Hippocratic era. Women's interpretation of physical symptoms were highly influenced by the "expert" knowledge of physicians whose task was not only to cure disease but also to explain it. See Nancy M. Theriot, "Women's Voices in the Nineteenth-Century Medical Discourse: A Step Toward Deconstructing Science," *Signs* 29 (1993): 1–31.

69. Nathaniel W. Emerson, M.D., "The Final Results in Operations for Myomata Uteri and Fibr-Myomata Uteri," *New England Medical Gazette*, (October 1903; reprint, CPP pamphlet, *Obstetrics/Gynecology* 159), 1–8.

70. Morantz-Sanchez, *Conduct Unbecoming*, 103, 107–108.

71. Theriot, "Women's Voices in the Nineteenth-Century Medical Discourse," 1–31.

72. Gail Pat Parsons argues that Victorian physicians prescribed similar treatment for male and female complaints, viewing both in terms of their reproductive systems. Rejecting the "conspiratorial" view of some scholars that nineteenth-century male physicians used deliberately punative therapeutics to keep women in their place, Parsons argues instead that physicians' misunderstood human sexuality. The state of medical knowledge, within the social/cultural context of Victorian America, guaranteed "equal treatment for all." While her point is well taken, she does not answer the central question of why "equal treatment" resulted in disproportionately more castrations of women. See "Equal Treatment for All: American Medical Remedies for Male Sexual Problems, 1850–1900," *Journal of the History of Medicine and Allied Sciences* 31, no. 1 (January 1977): 55–71.

73. Smith-Rosenberg and Rosenberg, "The Female Animal," (1984), 12–27. As Ornella Moscucci shows, gynecologists used two main models in explaining women's disease. Besides reflex theories, physicians also viewed the body as a closed energy system where the organs and mental faculties competed for a finite supply of energy. Depletion in one area resulted in exhaustion of the other (Edward Clarke's argument against intellectual work for women). See Ornella Moscucci, *The Science of Woman*, 102–108.

74. See Ludmilla Jordanova, *Sexual Visions: Images of Gender in Science and Medicine between the Eighteenth and Twentieth Centuries* (Madison: University of Wisconsin Press, 1989), in Theriot, "Women's Voices in the Nineteenth-Century Medical Discourse," *Signs* 29 (1993). Also see Susan E. Cayleff, "'Prisoners of Their Own Feebleness': Women, Nerves, and Western Medicine—A Historical Overview," *Social Science and Medicine* 26, no.12 (1988): 1199–1208.

75. As scholars have shown, the source for fueling the search for sex differences was a political one. Enlightenment thinkers, trying to reconcile the "natural" equality of all people with the higher authority of men, replaced Aristotelian and Christian teachings with the "objective" authority of science, countering the appeal to natural rights with proof of women's natural inequalities. Believing that women were ignoring their duties as wives and mothers at a time when Europe was losing population, the newly developed theory of sexual complementarity (where men and women were viewed not as physical and moral equals but complementary opposites) made inequalities seem natural while satisfying the need for a continued sexual division of labor. See Londa Schiebinger, *The Mind Has No Sex? Women in the Origins of Modern Science* (Cambridge: Harvard University Press, 1989), especially Chapters 6–8.

76. James W. Ward, M.D., "Radical Surgery of the Ovaries," *Pacific Coast Journal of Homoeopathy* 6, no. 10 (October 1898): 381.

77. Theriot, "Women's Voices," 13. See also Morantz-Sanchez, *Sympathy and Science* (1985), 221.

78. Theriot, "Women's Voices," 12.

79. Harriet Clisby, "Some Reminisences of Australia and America," WEIU Manuscript Collection. See also Sarah Deutsch, "Learning to Talk More Like a Man: Boston Women's Class-Bridging Organizations, 1870–1940," *American Historical Review* 97, no. 2 (April 1992): 379–404.

80. Brinkman, M.D., "The Relation of Homoeopathy to Gynaecology, 169–171.

81. Ibid., 172–173.

82. Morantz-Sanchez has identified a variety of reasons for women's absence in the field of gynecological surgery, including cultural assumptions that surgery was men's work, lack of access to developing male networks such as specialty societies, formalized courses of study, and internship and residency programs. See *Conduct Unbecoming a Woman*.

83. Florence N. Ward, M.D., "Conservative Surgery of the Ovary," *Pacific Coast Journal of Homoeopathy* 6, no. 11 (November 1898): 427.

84. Florence N. Ward, M.D., "Report of Three Years' Surgical Work," *Journal of the American Institute of Homoeopathy* 7 (April 1915): 1087–1095.

85. Florence N. Ward, "Therapeutics of Ovarian Diseases," *Pacific Coast Journal of Homoeopathy*" 7 (July 1898): 263–264.

Chapter 6   *Transformation of American Medicine*

1. "Minutes," *Transactions of the AIH* (1899), in William Rothstein, *American Physicians in the Nineteenth Century: From Sects to Science* (Baltimore: Johns Hopkins University Press, 1985), 245; and Naomi Rogers, "American Homeopathy Confronts Scientific Medicine," in *Culture, Knowledge, and Healing: Historical Perspectives of Homeopathic Medicine in Europe and North America*, ed. Robert Jutte, Guenter B. Risse, and John Woodward (Sheffield, UK: European Association for the History of Medicine and Health Publications, 1998), 47.

2. Holcombe, *Cresset* 1, no. 3 (January 1898), 39.

3. S. E. Chapman, "Homoeopathy the Science of Therapeutics," *Pacific Coast Journal of Homoeopathy* 6, no. 11 (November 1898): 422.

4. Burton J. Bledstein, *The Culture of Professionalism: The Middle Class and the Development of Higher Education in America* (New York: W. W. Norton & Co., 1976), xi.

5. Daniel M. Fox, *Health Policies and Health Politics: The British and American Experience, 1911–1965* (Princeton: Princeton University Press, 1986), 10; and Gerald E. Markowitz and David Rosner, "Doctors in Crisis: Medical Education and Medical Reform During the Progressive Era, 1895–1915," in *Health Care in America: Essays in Social History*, ed. Susan Reverby and David Rosner (Philadelphia: Temple University Press, 1979), 194. Analyses of the professionalization of medicine during the Progressive Era include: Ronald L. Numbers, "The Fall and Rise of the American Medical Profession," in *Sickness and Health in America: Readings in the History of Medicine and Public Health*, ed. Judith Walzer Leavitt and Ronald L. Numbers (Madison: University of Wisconsin Press, 1985), 185–196; Barbara Gutmann Rosenkrantz, "The Search for Professional Order in Nineteenth Century American Medicine," in *Sickness and Health in America*, 219–232; and Paul Starr, *The Social Transformation of American Medicine: The Rise of a Sovereign Profession and the Making of a Vast Industry* (New York: Basic Books, 1982), Chapter 3.

6. See Penina Migdal Glazer and Miriam Slater, *Unequal Colleagues: The Entrance of*

Women into the Professions, 1890–1940 (New Brunswick, N.J.: Rutgers University Press, 1987), especially Chapters 3 and 4; and Regina Morantz-Sanchez, *Sympathy and Science: Women Physicians in American Medicine* (New York: Oxford University Press, 1985), Chapter 9.

7. Starr, *The Social Transformation of American Medicine*, 107; and Samuel L. Baker, "Medical Licensing in America: An Early Liberal Reform," (Ph.D. diss., Department of Economics, Harvard University, 1977), cited in Rosenkrantz, *The Search for Professional Order*, 231, f. 22.

8. As scholars have shown, differences between osteopathy and organized medicine began to fade after 1930 when osteopathic colleges and hospitals de-emphasized distinctive osteopathic manipulative therapy in favor of pharmacotherapy. See Norman Gevitz, *The D.O.'s Osteopathic Medicine in America* (Baltimore: Johns Hopkins University Press, 1982), 88–98.

9. *Journal of the AIH* 17, no. 4 (April 1924): 355.

10. See Rogers, *An Alternative Path: The Making and Remaking of Hahnemann Medical College and Hospital of Philadelphia* (New Brunswick, N.J.: Rutgers University Press, 1998), 83–95; and "American Homeopathy Confronts Scientific Medicine," 31–64.

11. Rothstein, *American Physicians in the Nineteenth Century*, 321; and Martin Kaufman, *Homeopathy in America: The Rise and Fall of a Medical Heresy* (Baltimore: Johns Hopkins University Press, 1971), 153–155.

12. *Journal of the AMA* 43 (15 October 1904): 1158–1159, in Kaufman, *Homeopathy in America*, 155.

13. Hugo R. Arndt, "Report of the Field Secretary to the Board of Trustees, 1 December 1911," *Journal of the AIH* 4, no. 7 (January 1912): 913–915.

14. Hugo R. Arndt, "From the Field," *Journal of the AIH* 4, no. 5 (November 1911): 583.

15. Royal S. Copeland, M.D., "Effective Teaching in Our Colleges," *Journal of the AIH* 7, no. 3 (September 1914): 261.

16. James C. Wood, "The Relations of Homoeopathy to Allied Systems of Therapeutics," *Transactions of the AIH* (1899), 112–114: 117.

17. Editorial, *The Medical Visitor* 19 (August 1903): 776.

18. Editorial, *The Medical Visitor* (1 April 1902): 242.

19. I. T. Talbot, "Medical Education in the Homoeopathic Hospitals and Colleges of the United States," *Transactions of the World's Homoeopathic Congress*, 1893: 109.

20. Markowitz and Rosner, *Doctors in Crisis*, 186. The admission of women to the Johns Hopkins Medical School was influenced by monetary contributions to the institution from the National Woman's Fund Committee, especially a $300,000 donation from Dr. Mary Elizabeth Garrett. See Morantz-Sanchez, *Sympathy and Science*, 85–88.

21. Kenneth M. Ludmerer, *Learning to Heal: The Development of American Medical Education* (New York: Basic Books, 1985), 57–58, 63, 69.

22. Starr, *The Social Transformation of American Medicine*, 136–137.

23. Harris L. Coulter, *Divided Legacy: The Conflict Between Homoeopathy and the American Medical Association, Science and Ethics in American Medicine, 1800–1914*, 2d ed. (Berkeley, Calif.: North Atlantic Books, 1982), 444.

24. John Harley Warner, "The Fall and Rise of Professional Mystery: Epistemology, Authority, and the Emergence of Laboratory Medicine in Nineteenth-Century America," in *The Laboratory Revolution in Medicine*, ed. Andrew Cunningham and Perry Williams (Cambridge: Cambridge University Press, 1992), 115.

25. Marion Hunt, "From Childsaving to Pediatrics: A Case Study of Women's Role in

the Development of Saint Louis Children's Hospital, 1879–1925," (Ph.D. diss., Washington University, 1992), 107, 118–119.

26. Ibid., 149, 1–2, 86.

27. See Rosemary Stevens, *In Sickness and in Wealth: American Hospitals in the Twentieth Century* (New York: Basic Books, 1989), Chapter 2.

28. Percentages of women graduates were calculated from Winston Database. Between 1900 and 1910 women graduates numbered approximately 310.

29. See Morantz-Sanchez, *Sympathy and Science*, 249; and Mary Roth Walsh, *"Doctors Wanted: No Women Need Apply" Sexual Barriers in the Medical Profession, 1835–1975* (New Haven: Yale University Press, 1977), 178–206.

30. Schools that had closed by 1910 include: Cleveland Medical College (in existence from 1890 to 1897); Denver Homoeopathic Medical College and Hospital; Homoeopathic Medical College of Missouri in Saint Louis; Chicago Homoeopathic Medical College; Dunham Medical College in Chicago; and the College of Homoeopathic Medicine and Surgery of Kansas City University.

31. Morantz-Sanchez, *Sympathy and Science*, 261–263; and "Feminist Theory and Historical Practice: Rereading Elizabeth Blackwell," *History and Theory: Studies in the Philosophy of History*, Beiheft 31 (1992), 56–57. See also Charles Rosenberg, "The Therapeutic Revolution: Medicine, Meaning, and Social Change in Nineteenth-Century America," in *The Therapeutic Revolution: Essays on the Social History of American Medicine*, ed. C. Rosenberg and Morris Vogel (Philadelphia: University of Pennsylvania Press, 1979), 10–22.

32. Morantz-Sanchez, "Feminist Theory and Historical Practice: Rereading Elizabeth Blackwell," *History and Theory: Studies in the Philosophy of History*, Beiheft 31 (1992), 53–54; and Morantz-Sanchez, *Sympathy and Science*, 262–264.

33. Starr, *The Social Transformation of American Medicine*, 118.

34. For a discussion on coeducation's effect on women's medical schools, see Morantz-Sanchez, *Sympathy and Science*, 244–255.

35. *Journal of the AIH* 1, no. 11 (1909): 537.

36. Abraham Flexner, *Medical Education in the United States and Canada*, Bulletin No. 4 (New York: The Classics of Medicine Library, Special Edition 1990), 240, 271, 285, 214, 161.

37. Ibid., 161, 156, 162.

38. See James G. Burrow, *Organized Medicine in the Progressive Era: The Move Toward Monopoly* (Baltimore: Johns Hopkins University Press, 1977).

39. See E. Richard Brown, *Rockefeller Medicine Men: Medicine and Capitalism in America* (Berkeley: University of California Press, 1979).

40. Walsh, *"Doctors Wanted: No Women Need Apply,"* 198.

41. See "Complete Report of the Committee on Reorganization," In *History of the Reorganization of the Boston University School of Medicine*, (Boston: 1918), in Kaufman, *Homeopathy in America*, 171–172).

42. *Boston University Bulletin, 1919.*

43. See William H. Roberts, "Orthodoxy vs. Homeopathy: Ironic Developments Following the Flexner Report at the Ohio State University," *Bulletin of the History of Medicine* 60 (1986): 73–87.

44. Figures for women regulars and all medical students are from Morantz-Sanchez, *Sympathy and Science*, 249; and William G. Rothstein, *American Medical Schools and the Practice of Medicine* (New York: Oxford University Press, 1987), 143.

45. Numbers from Winston Database.

46. For example, see John S. Haller Jr. and Barbara Mason, *Forging a Medical Practice, 1884–1938 An Illinois Case Study: Wilber Price Armstrong* (Pearson Museum,

Southern Illinois University, 1997). As the authors show, Armstrong publicly identified himself as a "regular" physician in the 1900 Springfield city directory, yet continued to prescribe homeopathic remedies and maintained his affiliation with homeopathic medical societies throughout his professional career.

47. "The International Hahnemannian Association as a Factor for Good in the Homeopathic Profession," *Proceedings of the IHA* (1908): 14–15.

48. William Harvey King, ed., *History of Homoeopathy and Its Institutions in America* 2 (New York: Lewis Publishing Co., 1905), 427–429.

49. Rachel Tenney, "New Medical Opportunities," *Woman's Medical Journal* 1, no. 8 (August 1893): 167.

50. King, ed. *History of Homoeopathy* 2 (1905), 430–432.

51. Tenney, "New Medical Opportunities," 167.

52. Flexner, *Medical Education in the United States and Canada*, 214.

53. Ibid., 160. Others included Southwestern in Louisville; Pulte in Cincinnati; Atlantic in Baltimore (aka Southern Homoeopathic Medical College and Hospital); and homeopathic schools in Detroit and Kansas City.

54. King, ed., *History of Homoeopathy* 3 (1905), 120.

55. Ibid, 2:431.

56. "Minutes of the Board of Directors," (19 November 1891), *Philadelphia Post-Graduate School of Homeopathics.*

57. Based on recent research by John S. Haller Jr., see also Julian Winston, "A Modern Biography of James Tyler Kent," *The American Homeopath* 2 (1995): 9–11.

58. "Minutes of the Board of Directors," (1 July 1896), Philadelphia Post-Graduate School of Homeopathics.

59. Samuel Hahnemann, *Organon of Medicine* (1833), trans. R. E. Dudgeon, from the 5th ed., rev. and enl. 6th ed. trans. William Boericke (reprint, New Delhi: B. Jain Publishers , 1996), 33–35. In the 6th ed. of the *Organon*, Hahnemann replaced the term "vital force" with "vital principle," and referred to "force" as "energy." The date of Hahnemann's last manuscript of the *Organon* is estimated as 1842. See page 19.

60. James Tyler Kent, *Lectures on Homoeopathic Philosophy* (1900; reprint, Berkeley, Calif.: North Atlantic Books, 1979), 68–69, 73.

61. Stuart Close, "The Identity of Hahnemann's 'Vital Force' with the Subconscious Mind," *Homoeopathic Recorder* 38, no. 5 (15 May 1923): 311.

62. R. Del Mas, "Pathology vs. the Hahnemannian Homoeopath," *The Homoeopathician* 1, no. 3 (March 1912).

63. Winston, "A Modern Biography of James Tyler Kent," 9. With his emphasis on psychological as well as physiological history and function, Kent's constitutional "types" differed from constitutional practitioners of the early twentieth century whose profiles included morphological and biological characteristics such as body measurements and results of blood and urine analysis. See Sarah W. Tracy, "George Draper and American Constitutional Medicine, 1916–1946: Reinventing the Sick Man," *Bulletin of the History of Medicine* 66, no. 1 (spring 1992): 53–89.

64. Kent, *Lectures on Homoeopathic Philosophy*, 24.

65. In 1900 Kent relocated the Post-Graduate School to Dunham Medical College in Chicago and became dean of that institution. The last class to graduate was in 1903, one year after the merger of Dunham and Hering.

66. WMCP graduates included Rosalie Stankowitz, Mary Ives, Mary Branson, Mary K. Jackson, Lydia W. Stokes, Amelia Hess, and Julia Loos.

67. "Minutes of the Board of Directors," (20 May 1897) *Philadelphia Post-Graduate School of Homeopathics.*

68. *The Homoeopathician* 1, no. 1 (January 1912): 12–15. *The Homoeopathician* was published from 1912 to 1916, and little is known about the society after this time.

It may have dissolved when the journal ceased publication. Women founders and graduates included Alice H. Bassett (Boston), Fredericka E. Gladwin (Philadelphia), Margaret C. Lewis (Philadelphia), Julia Loos (Harrisburg, Pa.), and Carrie E. Newton (Maine).

69. "Homoeopathy vs. Homoeopathicians," *Medical Century* 4, no. 2 (January 1896): 46–78.
70. Stuart Close, Editorial, *Homeopathic Recorder* 38, no. 2 (15 February 1923): 81.
71. "Science and Art of Medicine," *Homoeopathic Recorder* 4 (15 April 1923): 138, 169.
72. *Homoeopathic Recorder* 9 (15 September 1923).
73. *Homoeopathic Physician* 7 (1887), 145, in Coulter, *Divided Legacy*, 443.
74. Total numbers in the IHA were 138 men and 34 women. There were approximately 2,203 men in the AIH and 309 women. Numbers are hand counted from the *International Homoeopathic Medical Directory, 1911–1912*, (London: Homoeopathic Publishing Co.), and *Proceedings of the IHA* (1910), 219–235.
75. Various *Proceedings of the IHA* from 1897 to 1915.
76. T. J. Jackon Lears, *No Place of Grace: Antimodernism and the Transformation of American Culture, 1880–1920* (Chicago: University of Chicago Press, 1981), 42–47.
77. Ibid., 34–38.
78. Ibid., 142–143; 175–176; 316–318.
79. Ibid., xi.
80. Ibid., xv, xvi.
81. Kent, *Lectures on Homoeopathic Philosophy*, 50–51.
82. Ibid., 17, 24, 85. From "lazzaro" or leper, lazaretto defined an institution or hospital for people with contagious diseases.
83. "A Scientific Basis for Homoeopathy," *Cresset* 1, no. 5 (March 1898), 67.
84. Charles Edmund Fisher, M.D., "The Practical Side of Homeopathy," *Medical Century* 8, no. 3 (1 March 1900): 88.
85. Bureau of Homoeopathic Philosophy," *Proceedings of the IHA* (1921): 69. As one scholar notes, rather than a linear series of truths awaiting inevitable recognition, a particular theory or innovation becomes "scientific" only when demonstrated to be a step on the path toward what is presently recognized as "true." See S.E.D. Shortt, "Physicians, Science, and Status: Issues in the Professionalization of Anglo-American Medicine in the Nineteenth Century," *Medical History* 27 (March 1983): 51–68.
86. Ella A. Jennings, "A Plea for Homeopathy," *Medical Century* 2, no. 8 (15 April 1894): 175.
87. *Homoeopathy: A Pamphlet for the People* (Cambridge, Mass.: Louis F. Weston Press, 1900).
88. Ibid., 9–14.
89. Morantz-Sanchez, "Feminist Theory and Historical Practice: Rereading Elizabeth Blackwell," *History and Theory*, 61, 51, 59.

Chapter 7 *Struggle for Survival*

1. Elinore Peebles interview by Louise Woofenden, 13 November 1986 and 1 January 1987).
2. Only the New York Homoeopathic Medical College and Hahnemann University in Philadelphia were in existence at this time. Examples of hospitals dropping homeopathic designations include Buffalo Homoeopathic Hospital, which became the Millard Filmore Hospital. See *Journal of the AIH* 17, no. 2 (February

1924): 185. Many converted their staffs from homeopathic doctors to academic physicians trained in "scientific" medical schools. See Marion Hunt, "From Child-saving to Pediatrics: A Case Study of Women's Role in the Development of Saint Louis Children's Hospital, 1879–1925" (Ph.D. diss., Washington University, 1992). Homeopaths in Boston around this time were struggling to maintain home-opathy in the hospital associated with the homoeopathic medical school at Boston University. However, in a few locations, homeopathic hospitals received sufficient financial support to upgrade their facilities substantially. For example, the Rochester Homoeopathic Hospital raised $600,000 for construction of a new five-story pavilion. See *Journal of AIH* 17, no. 5 (May 1925): 466.

3. Peebles interview, 27.
4. Peebles interview, 28.
5. Richard Moskowitz as cited in Julian Winston, *The Faces of Homoeopathy: An Illustrated History of the First 200 Years* (Tawa, NZ: Great Awk Publishing, 1999), 343.
6. "Editorial," *Homoeopathic Recorder* 38, no. 4 15 April 1923, 138. The selection of the "proper" homeopathic remedy was (and is) believed to affect the whole person constitutionally and psychosomatically rather than singular organs or functions.
7. "Editorial," *Homoeopathic Recorder* 38, no. 5 15 May 1923, 273–274.
8. Dr. Mary E. Hanks, interview by Mary Ware Dennett, Chicago, 11 February 1927, 4. All reports of interviews cited in this chapter are located in the National Center for Homeopathy Archives, box 56.
9. *Journal of the AIH* 7, no. 1 (July 1914): 1–13; and *Proceedings of the IHA, 1919–1920*: 16–17, 222–226.
10. James C. Wood, "Modernism vs. Fundamentalism in Medicine," *Journal of the AIH* 17, no. 3 (March 1924): 269–270.
11. *Journal of the AIH* 17, no. 1 (January 1924): 75.
12. *Journal of the AIH* 17, no. 3 (March 1924): 276–277.
13. *Journal of the AIH* 17, no. 1 (January 1924): 75.
14. *Journal of the AIH* 4, no. 5 (November 1911): 584.
15. *Journal of the AIH* 2, no. 5 (May 1910): 307.
16. *Journal of the AIH* 17, no. 5 (May 1924): 454.
17. Ibid.
18. Ibid.
19. *Journal of the AIH* 17, no. 6 (June 1924): 71–72.
20. Ibid.
21. *Journal of the AIH* 20, no. 3.
22. Dr. Mary E. Hanks, interview by Mary Ware Dennett, Chicago, 11 February 1927.
23. See John S. Haller Jr. and Barbara Mason, *Forging a Medical Practice, 1884–1938, An Illinois Case Study: Wilber Price Armstrong* (Pearson Museum, Southern Illinois University, 1997).
24. The prevalence of joint membership is evidenced in the 1924 resolution adopted by members of the IHA barring from office anyone affiliated with "any society in the AMA." According to one source, several officers of national, state, and local homeopathic societies were members of orthodox organizations. See *Proceedings of the IHA* (1924), 5, 19. Wesselhoeft later became president of the Massachusetts Medical Society. See obituary in the *Journal of the American Medical Association* (JAMA) 184, no. 6 (11 May 1963): 511–512.
25. Examples include Mary Ware Dennett's interviews with Dr. Cornelia Chase Brant, New York City, 28 November 1925; Dr. Morris Elting Gore, New York City, 27 January 1926; and Dr. John Hutchinson, New York City, 1 December 1925.
26. Dr. Margaret Lewis, interview by MWD, Philadelphia, 9 December 1925.
27. Dr. Cornelia Chase Brant interview by MWD, New York City, 28 November 1925.

28. Dr. Morris Elting Gore, interview by MWD, N.J., 27 January 1926.
29. Dr. Alice Parkhurst, interview by MWD, Baltimore, November 1926.
30. Dr. Stella Q. Root, interview by MWD, Stamford, Conn., 29 March 1926, AFH Archives.
31. Dr. Fredericka Moore; Dr. Susan M. Coffin; Dr. Mary R. Lakeman, interviews by MWD, Boston, 25 March 1927.
32. Guernsey P. Waring, "Foundations of Homoeopathy," *Proceedings of the IHA* (1910), 5, and Julia Green to Julia Loos, 5 August 1920, *Digest of Correspondence* (31 August 1921) 4 NCH Archives, box 7.
33. "Certificate of Incorporation," and "Trustees of the American Foundation for Homoeopathy," NCH Archives, box 6. Trustees were Alonzo E. Austin (1868–1948), New York City; Cyrus M. Boger (1861–1935), Parkersburg, W.Va.; George E. Dienst (1858–1932), Aurora, Ill.; Herbert A. Roberts (1868–1950), Derby, Conn.); Fredericka E. Gladwin (1856–1931), Philadelphia; Julia C. Loos (1869–1929), Baltimore; and Julia M. Green (1871–1963), Washington, D.C. Lay trustee George E. Fleming was vice president of the Union Trust Company in Washington, D. C.
34. Ibid.
35. See Chapter 4 on women's fundraising activities for homeopathic hospitals.
36. Julia Minerva Green (JMG) to Trustees, 13 June 1923.
37. *Minutes to Meeting of AFH Trustees*, 4 July 1923.
38. *Proceedings of the IHA* June 1930: 24–26.
39. For a discussion of the Society of Homoeopathicians, see Chapter 6.
40. "high-potency cranks" was a common epithet used by progressive homeopaths to describe traditionalists whose interpretation of Hahnemann's *Organon* led to prescribing extremely diluted remedies.
41. Julia Green, (report to Wellesley class secretary, n.d.) as cited in Kay Vargo, "Julia Minerva Green, M.D.: A Master Prescriber," n.p. Vargo, a longtime secretary to the AFH and personal friend of Green's, generously provided me with a copy of her unpublished manuscript, the source of the above biographical information on Green.
42. Reformer and suffrage activist Clemence Lozier founded the first women's homeopathic school in the United States. See Chapter 3.
43. See Dorte Staudt, "The Role of Laymen in the History of German Homeopathy," in *Culture, Knowledge, and Healing: Historical Perspectives of Homeopathic Medicine in Europe and North America*, ed. Robert Jutte, Guenter B. Risse, and John Woodward (Sheffield, UK: European Association for the History of Medicine and Health Publications, 1998), 199–215.
44. Elizabeth B. Magruder, "Some Notes on the Early History of the Homoeopathic Laymen's League of Washington, D. C., (30 June 1936), *Record*.
45. "Addendum Adjourned Meeting," 16 June 1925, 1.
46. Constance M. Chen, *"The Sex Side of Life": Mary Ware Dennett's Pioneering Battle for Birth Control and Sex Education* (New York: New Press, 1996), 135–136.
47. Dennett called Margaret Sanger's approach to providing women with access to birth control information through physicians a type of "class legislation." Believing that despite laws, the rich would always have access to birth control, Dennett insisted birth control information and devices belonged in the hands of women rather than the mostly male medical establishment. Dennett also disagreed with Sanger's efforts to overturn laws restricting birth control in individual states, rather than attacking the problem at the national level. See Chen, *"The Sex Side of Life,"* 213–214.
48. As a child in Boston, Dennett was a patient of Dr. William Wesselhoeft. See Mary Ware Dennett (MWD) to JMG, 21 April 1925.

49. MWD to Julia Green, 21 April 1925.
50. Chen, "*The Sex Side of Life*," 160.
51. Ibid., 50, 16, 23, 246.
52. Ibid., 175–176.
53. Ibid., 227.
54. Ibid., 229, 269. In 1929, Dennett was indicted for violation of U.S. Criminal Code prohibiting the distribution of "obscene" material via the United States Postal Service.
55. MWD, AFH/IHA meeting, 26 June 1925, 169.
56. For discussions of the various strands of antimodernism, see T. J. Jackson Lears, *No Place of Grace: Antimodernism and the Transformation of American Culture, 1880–1920* (Chicago: University of Chicago Press, 1981).
57. Ibid.
58. MWD to Julia Minerva Green, "Lincoln's Birthday," 1930.
59. Mary Ware Dennett Defense Committee, "Sex Education—Freedom or Censorship," (public hearing 21 May 1929), MWD Papers, folder 484, box 27, cited in Chen, "*The Sex Side of Life*," 247, f778.
60. MWD meeting report to AFH/IHA, 26 June 1925, 169.
61. See *Greater than the Parts: Holism in Biomedicine, 1920–1950*, ed. Christopher Lawrence and George Weisz (New York: Oxford University Press, 1998). As the contributors to this book show, holism has a variety of related but distinct meanings. The popularity of naturopathy and homeopathy in France, Germany, the United States, and to a lesser extent in Great Britain, influenced several forms of ideological holism within mainstream medicine. See Chapter 4, George Weisz, "A Moment of Synthesis: Medical Holism in France between the Wars," 71.
62. MWD to JMG, Boston, 19 March 1927, 2.
63. Ibid., 3.
64. MWD to JMG, 25 July 1925.
65. JMG to MWD, 31 July 1925.
66. MWD to JMG, 19 July 1925.
67. MWD to JMG, 14 August 1925, 2.
68. MWD interviews with Dr. John Hutchinson, 1 December 1925; Dr. E. Wallace Madadam, 10 November 1925; Dr. Rudolph Rabe, 14 November 1925; Dr. Morris Elting Gore, 27 January 1926; and Dr. Margaret Lewis, 9 December 1925.
69. Dr. Frederick M. Dearborn, interview by MWD, NYC, 21 January 1926. See also Martin Kaufman, *Homeopathy in America: The Rise and Fall of a Medical Heresy* (Baltimore: Johns Hopkins University Press, 1971), 175.
70. MWD to JMG, 16 January 1926.
71. MWD to JMG, 18 January 1926.
72. MWD to JMG, 16 January 1926.
73. Dr. Alice Butler, interview by MWD, Cleveland, 25 May 1926. Butler was a 1900 graduate of the homeopathic medical school at Boston University.
74. Dr. Jennie Medley, interview by MWD, Philadelphia, 5 February 1926.
75. Dr. Fredericka Moore, Dr. Susan M. Coffin, and Dr. Mary R. Lakeman, joint interview by MWD, Boston, 25 March 1927. Moore, Coffin, and Lakeman were graduates of the homeopathic medical school at BU in 1910, 1905, and 1895, respectively. Their careers in public health were typical of the general connection of women physicians with social medicine in the 1920s even as its "glitter" faded with the decline of public enthusiasm for social reform after World War I. See Regina Morantz-Sanchez, *Sympathy and Science: Women Physicians in American Medicine* (New York: Oxford University Press, 1985), 309.
76. Martin Kaufman, *Homeopathy in America*, 171–172.
77. Dr. Alice H. Bassett, interview by MWD, Boston, 11 February 1926.

78. Ronald L. Numbers, "The Fall and Rise of the American Medical Profession," in *Sickness and Health in America: Readings in the History of Medicine and Public Health*, ed. Judith Walzer Leavitt and Ronald L. Numbers (Madison: University of Wisconsin Press, 1985), 185–196. See also Benjamin C. Woodbury, M.D., "The Healing Power of Nature: 'The Invisible Increment,'" *Homoeopathic Recorder* 35, no. 10 (15 October 1920): 454–455. Homeopathy lost its "edge" to the newer alternatives in other cities as well. For example, see Thomas Neville Bonner, *Medicine in Chicago, 1850–1950: A Chapter in the Social and Scientific Development of a City*, 2d ed. (Urbana and Chicago: University of Illinois Press, 1991).
79. Woodbury, "The Healing Power of Nature," 454–455.
80. Lawrence and Weisz, "Medical Holism: The Context," in *Greater than the Parts*, 5.
81. T. H. Carmichael, M.D., *Homoeopathic Recorder* 36, no. 8 (15 August 1921): 336.
82. Dr. Stella Q. Root, interview by MWD, Stamford, Conn., 29 March 1926. Root discussed Wesselhoeft in her meeting with Dennett.
83. For example, see Dr. Bina Seymour, interview by MWD, Boston, 24 February 1926; and Dr. William Jefferson Guernsey, interview by MWD, Philadelphia, 11 March 1926.
84. Stella Q. Root interview, 2–3.
85. Dr. Elizabeth Wright, "Confidential for Dr. Green," interview by MWD, 5 April 1927.
86. *Minutes to the Semi-Annual Meeting of the Board of Trustees of the AFH*, 1 July 1927: 29–30.
87. Sarah Nielsen, "Pioneering Women Homeopaths," *The American Homeopath* 3 (1997): 32–33.
88. The remedy refers to carbonate of ammonia (an alkaline compound of nitrogen and hydrogen) at the 10,000th dilution or potency.
89. Elizabeth Wright Hubbard, "On First Attempting to Prescribe Homeopathically," in *Homoeopathy as Art and Science*, ed. Dr. Maesimund B. Panos and Della DesRosiers (Beaconsfield, Bucks, England: Beaconsfield Publishers, 1990), 265.
90. Dr. Alice H. Bassett, interview by MWD, Boston, 11 February 1926.
91. Dr. Elizabeth Wright, interview by MWD, Boston, 26 February 1926.
92. Dr. Vesta Charlotte Wandell, interview by MWD, Oak Park, Ill., 27 January 1927.
93. Dr. Mary E. Hanks, interview by MWD, Chicago, 11 February 1927.
94. Dr. Alice Butler, interview by MWD, Cleveland, 25 May 1926.
95. Dr. Julia C. Strawn, Dr. Lillian Thompson, and Dr. Frances Gage Hulbert, interview by MWD, Chicago, 20 January 1927.
96. Dr. Mary E. Hanks, interview by MWD, Chicago, 11 February 1927.
97. Based on one hundred interviews.
98. Mrs. C. M. Sigler, Harrisburg, Pa, 19 March 1926; Mrs. B. F. Snavely, Lancaster, Pa, 20 March 1926; and Mr. Louis Musil, New York City, 6 January 1926.
99. Mrs. C. M. Sigler, Harrisburg, Pa., 19 March 1926; Mrs. Frank A. Hall, Montclair, N.J., 1 February 1926; Mrs. William S. Hallowell, Philadelphia, 9 December 1926; Captain Harrison A. Bispham, Philadelphia, 11 December 1925; and Mrs. John S. Reed, Waltham, Mass., 17 March 1927.
100. Mrs. Leopold Auer, 24 November 1925.
101. Mr. and Mrs. Walter A. Sheriffs and Mrs. R. J. Gaudy, Winnetka, Ill., 2 February 1927.
102. Mr. John S. Dove Jr., Philadelphia, 1 March 1926; and Bruce Walter, Pittsburgh, Pa., 20 April 1926.
103. Mrs. J. A. L. Waddell, New York City, 13 March (no year).
104. Alma Hiller, New York City, 10 May 1926; and Mr. Decatur M. Sawyer, Montclair, N.J., 6 January 1927.
105. Mr. and Mrs. Walter A. Sheriffs and Mrs. R. J. Gaudy, Winnetka, Ill. 2 February

1927; Edward C. Bostock, Philadelphia, 17 December 1925; and Mr. Hermann L. Grote, Pittsburgh, Pa., 17 April 1926.
106. Mr. and Mrs. Harry Parkhurst, Baltimore, Md., 7 November 1926.
107. Albert D. Henderson, Chicago and Glenview, Ill., 17 February 1927.
108. Bryn Athyn report by MWD, 16 December 1925; and 6 March 1926, AFH, box 56; and report of meeting at the home of Rev. William L. Worcester, Cambridge, Mass., 4 April 1927. By "real homeopaths," the author assumes Moses was referring to Hahnemannian patients.
109. Mrs. George D. Pike, Boston, 13 April 1927; and Dr. Julia Strawn, Chicago, 18 February 1927.
110. MWD to JMG, 12 April 1926; and JMG to MWD, 10 April 1926.
111. Rosemary Stevens, *In Sickness and in Wealth: American Hospitals in the Twentieth Century* (New York: Basic Books, 1989), 129.
112. Dr. C. Louis Olds, Bryn Athyn, Pa., 11 December 1925.
113. JMG to MWD, 17 September 1926.
114. MWD to JMG, 25 November 1926.
115. E. Richard Brown, *Rockefeller Medicine Men: Medicine and Capitalism in America* (Berkeley: University of California Press, 1979), 193–194.
116. Mary Ware Dennett, "Patient Summaries."
117. *Minutes to the Meeting of the Board of Trustees of the AFH*, 6 December 1925; and *Minutes to the Semi-Annual Meeting of the Board of Trustees*, 1 July 1927: 4.
118. See for example, Dr. Alice H. Bassett, interview by Mary Ware Dennett, Boston, 11 February 1926; and Dr. Walter Gray Crump, interview by MWD, 13 January 1926.
119. MWD to JMG, 6 January 1926.
120. Dr. Alice H. Basset, interview by MWD, Boston, 11 February 1926.
121. Linda Gordon, *Woman's Body, Woman's Right: Birth Control in America* (New York: Penguin Books, rev. 1990), 281.
122. *Minutes to the Semi-Annual Meeting of the Board of Trustees of the AFH*, 1 July 1927, 36.
123. Morantz-Sanchez, *Sympathy and Science*, 336, 356.
124. *Minutes to the Semi-Annual Meeting of the Board of Trustees of the AFH*, 1 July 1927: 36, 43, 62–70.
125. Ibid., 4.
126. *Minutes to the Meeting of the Board of Trustees of the AFH*, 24 January 1928.
127. *Minutes to the Meeting of the Board of Trustees of the AFH*, December 1927.
128. Morantz-Sanchez, *Sympathy and Science*, 311.
129. Sarah Nielsen, "Pioneering Women Homeopaths" 3 (1997), 33.
130. Morantz-Sanchez, *Sympathy and Science*, 320.
131. Julia Green to Dr. Lindeman, 1957, in Katherine Vargo, "Julia Minerva Green, M.D., A Master Prescriber," (n.d.).
132. The two most prominent were the *Journal of the AIH* and *The Homoeopathic Recorder*, publication of the IHA.
133. Inez Philbrick, *Medical Woman's Journal* (1929), cited in Morantz-Sanchez, *Sympathy and Science*, 317.

Epilogue　　*Twentieth-Century Transformation and Rebirth*

1. Naomi Rogers makes this argument in "Women and Sectarian Medicine," in *Women, Health, and Medicine in America*, ed. Rima D. Apple (New Brunswick, N.J.: Rutgers University Press, 1992), 284.
2. Osler to Vaughan, Baltimore, 16 February 1895, Vaughan Letters, as cited in John Harley Warner, "Orthodoxy and Otherness: Homeopathy and Regular Medicine

in Nineteenth-Century America," in *Culture, Knowledge, and Healing: Historical Perspectives of Homeopathy Medicine in Europe and North America*, ed. Robert Jutte, Guenter B. Risse and John Woodward (Sheffield, UK: European Association for the History of Medicine and Health Publications, 1998), 20.

3. *Johns Hopkins University Medical Department Tenth Annual Catalog and Announcements, 1902–1903* (Baltimore: Johns Hopkins University Press, 1902).

4. *Twilight Sleep Scrapbook 2*, Eliza T. Ransom Papers.

5. See Appendix B.

6. The name of the newspaper of this photocopied news article is missing. Only the date remains (26 June 1904), Eliza T. Ransom Papers.

7. Franklin H. Martin, *Fifty Years of Medicine and Surgery: An Autobiographical Sketch* (Chicago: Surgical Publishing Co., 1934), 417.

8. Naomi Rogers, "The Public Face of Homoeopathy: Politics, the Public, and Alternative Medicine in the United States, 1900–1940," in *Patients in the History of Homoeopathy*, ed. Martin Dinges (Sheffield, UK: European Association for the History of Medicine and Health Publications, 2000), 351–371.

9. Harry M. Marks, *The Progress of Experiment: Science and Therapeutic Reform in the United States, 1900–1990* (Cambridge: Cambridge University Press, 1997), 19–22.

10. Eugene Underhill Jr., "Traditional Medicine and Homoeopathy," *Homoeopathic Recorder* 47, no. 4 (April 1932): 258–259.

11. Marks, *The Progress of Experiment*, 37–38.

12. Ibid., 61.

13. Ibid., 37. Also see E. Richard Brown, *Rockefeller Medicine Men: Medicine and Capitalism in America* (Berkeley: University of California Press, 1979); and Naomi Rogers, *Dirt and Disease: Polio Before FDR* (New Brunswick, N.J.: Rutgers University Press, 1958), 72–105.

14. Laura B. Hurd, "Homoeopathic Medication of Lingering Conditions," *Journal of the AIH* 21, no. 7 (July 1928): 609–612.

15. *The Layman Speaks* 3, no. 12 (September 1950): 332–336.

16. E. Underhill Jr., *Proceedings of the IHA, 1931 and The Homoeopathic Recorder* 47, no. 4 (April 1932): 258–259.

17. Subcommittee on Constitutional Rights," *The Layman Speaks* 8, no. 10 (October 1955): 361; and Alfred Pulford, M.D., "The Modern Medical Prevention Racket, *The Homoeopathic Recorder* (March 1937): 120, 127; and Underhill Jr., Editorial, *The Homoeopathic Recorder* 60, no. 15 (May 1941).

18. Elizabeth Wright Hubbard, President's Page, *The Layman Speaks* 13, no. 8 (August 1960); reprint *Journal of the American Institute of Homoeopathy/The Homoeopathic Recorder* 54, no. 5 and no. 6 (May–June 1960).

19. For an overview of various strands of the 1960s counterculture, see Todd Gitlin, *The Sixties: Years of Hope, Days of Rage* (New York: Bantam Books, 1987, 1993); and Stewart Burns, *The Social Movements of the 1960s: Searching for Democracy* (Boston: Twayne Publication, 1990).

20. Helen Pohlmer to Kay Vargo, 13 February 1971, folder: New York Laymen's League, AFH, box 51.

21. Lesley Doyal, "Women, Health, and the Sexual Division of Labor: A Case Study of the Women's Health Movement in Britain," in *Women's Health, Politics, and Power: Essays on Sex/Gender, Medicine, and Public Health*, ed. Elizabeth Fee and Nancy Krieger (Amityville, N.Y.: Baywood Publishing Co., 1994), 61–76. See also Anne Taylor Kirschmann, "Making Friends for Pure Homoeopathy," and Amy Bix, "Engendering Alternatives: Women's Health-Care Choices and Feminist Medical Rebellions," in *The Politics of Healing: Essays in the Twentieth-Century History of North American Alternative Medicine* (New York: Routledge Press, forthcoming).

22. Massachusetts nurse practitioner Lauren Fox remembered feeling a definite "woman's connection" from the beginning of her involvement in homeopathic medicine in the early 1970s. Her Cape Cod homeopathic study group was led by a woman (eventually Fox assumed the position), and was comprised mostly of mothers of young children.

23. Lisa Harvey, M.D., telephone interview by author, 17 August 2000. Harvey received a BS degree from West Virginia University in 1975 and her M.D. degree from Wake Forest University in 1979. She currently practices medicine in western Massachusetts, focusing on family health care and homeopathy.

24. Lia Bello, R.N., telephone interview by author, 17 November 2000. Bello is currently a family nurse practitioner certified in classical homeopathy with a practice in Questa, New Mexico.

25. See for example T. J. Jackson Lears, *No Place of Grace: Antimodernism and the Transformation of American Culture, 1880–1920* (Chicago: University of Chicago Press, 1981); and Christopher Lasch, *The True and Only Heaven: Progress and its Critics* (New York: W. W. Norton & Co., 1991).

26. For a concise and colorful history of late-twentieth-century holistic healing see James C. Whorton, *Nature Cures: The History of Alternative Medicine in America*, (New York: Oxford University Press, 2002). Medical journal articles detailing late-twentieth-century trends in alternative therapeutics include David M. Eisenberg, et.al., "Unconventional Medicine in the United States: Prevalence, Costs, and Patterns of Use," *New England Journal of Medicine* (1993): 328, 246–252, and "Trends in Alternative Medicine Use in the United States, 1990–1997," *Journal of the American Medical Association* (1998) 280: 1569–1575; and Wayne B. Jonas, "Alternative Medicine—Learning from the Past, Examining the Present, Advancing to the Future," *Journal of the American Medical Association* (1998) 280: 1616–1618.

27. Julia M. Green, Obituary, *The Pacific Coast Homeopathic Bulletin* 12, no. 1 (January 1964; reprint *Washington Post*, 12 December 1963.

Manuscript Sources

Alumni Medical Library, Boston University School of Medicine. Boston, Mass. Boston University School of Medicine Collection; Massachusetts Homeopathic Hospital Collection.

Archives and Special Collections on Women in Medicine and Homeopathy, Drexel University College of Medicine. Philadelphia, Pa. American Medical Women's Association Historical Collection; Post-Graduate School of Homeopathics of Philadelphia Files; Thomas L. Bradford Scrapbooks, Thirty-five Volumes; Woman's Medical College of Pennsylvania Alumnae Files; Women Physicians Collection.

Arthur M. and Elizabeth Schlesinger Library, Radcliffe College. Cambridge, Mass. Eliza Taylor Ransom Papers; Martha George Ripley Papers; Women's Educational and Industrial Union Collection.

Cleveland Health Sciences Library, Historical Division. Cleveland, Ohio. Cleveland Homeopathic College Papers; Minutes of the Faculty of the Western College of Homoeopathy, 1867–1868.

College of Physicians of Philadelphia. Philadelphia, Pa. Homeopathic Pamphlet Collection; Lisabeth M. Holloway Collection.

Francis A. Countway Library of Medicine, Harvard University. Boston, Mass. Massachusetts Medical Society Collection; Women in Medicine Collection.

Historical Society of Pennsylvania. Philadelphia, Pa. Harriet Judd Sartain Papers. Samuel Sartain Collection.

Miami County Historical Society. Troy, Ohio. M. Belle Brown Papers.

National Center for Homeopathy. Alexandria, Va. American Foundation for Homeopathy Collection, including Julia M. Green Correspondence; Mary Ware Dennett Correspondence; Minutes to the Board of Trustees; Reports of Interviews and Meetings.

New York Academy of Medicine. New York City, N.Y. *Cressett*; Minutes of Alumnae Association; New York Medical College and Hospital for Women. Reports.

Ohio Historical Society. Columbus, Ohio. Janney Family Papers.

Syracuse University Archives. Syracuse, N.Y. The Comfort Family Papers.

Selected Bibliography

Abrahams, Harold J. *Extinct Medical Schools of Nineteenth-Century Philadelphia.* Philadelphia: University of Pennsylvania Press, 1966.

Ahlstrom, Sydney E. *A Religious History of the American People.* New Haven: Yale University Press, 1972.

Atwater, Edward C. "The Physicians of Rochester, New York, 1860–1910: A Study in Professional History 2." *Bulletin of the History of Medicine* 51 (1977).

Banner, Lois W. *American Beauty.* New York: Alfred A. Knopf, 1983.

———. *Elizabeth Cady Stanton: A Radical for Woman's Rights.* Boston: Little, Brown & Co., 1980.

Barlow, William, and David O. Powell. "Homeopathy and Sexual Equality: The Controversy over Coeducation at Cincinnati's Pulte Medical College, 1873–1879." In *Women and Health in America: Historical Readings.* Edited by Judith Walzer Leavitt. Madison: University of Wisconsin Press, 1984.

Beckwith, D. H. *History of the Cleveland Homoeopathic College from 1850–1880.* Cleveland, Ohio, n.d.

Bell, Whitfield J. Jr. *The College of Physicians of Philadelphia.* Science History Publications, 1987.

Berliner, Howard S. *A System of Scientific Medicine: Philanthropic Foundations in the Flexner Era.* New York and London: Tavistock Publications, 1985.

Bledstein, Burton J. *The Culture of Professionalism: The Middle Class and the Development of Higher Education in America.* New York: W. W. Norton & Co., 1976.

Bonner, Thomas Neville. *To the Ends of the Earth: Women's Search for Education in Medicine.* Cambridge: Harvard University Press, 1992.

———. *Medicine in Chicago, 1850–1950: A Chapter in the Social and Scientific Development of a City.* 2d ed. Urbana and Chicago: University of Illinois Press, 1991.

Brown, E. Richard. *Rockefeller Medicine Men: Medicine and Capitalism in America.* Berkeley: University of California Press, 1979.

Bullough, Vern, and Martha Voght. "Women, Menstruation, and Nineteenth-Century Medicine." In *Women and Health in America: Historical Readings.* Edited by Judith Walzer Leavitt. Madison: University of Wisconsin Press, 1984.

Burrow, James G. *Organized Medicine in the Progressive Era: The Move Toward Monopoly.* Baltimore: Johns Hopkins University Press, 1977.

Bynum, W. F. *Science and the Practice of Medicine in the Nineteenth Century.* Cambridge: Cambridge University Press, 1994.

———, and Roy Porter, eds. *Medical Fringe and Medical Orthodoxy, 1750–1850*. London: Croom Helm, 1987.

Cassedy, James H. *American Medicine and Statistical Thinking, 1800–1860*. Cambridge: Harvard University Press, 1984.

Cayleff, Susan E. "'Prisoners of their own Feebleness': Women, Nerves, and Western Medicine—A Historical Overview." *Social Science and Medicine* 26, no. 12 (1988).

———. *Wash and Be Healed: The Water-Cure Movement and Women's Health*. Philadelphia: Temple University Press, 1987.

Chen, Constance M. *"The Sex Side of Life": Mary Ware Dennett's Pioneering Battle for Birth Control and Sex Education*. New York: The New Press, 1996.

Cott, Nancy F. *The Grounding of Modern Feminism*. New Haven: Yale University Press, 1987.

Coulter, Harris L. *Divided Legacy: The Conflict Between Homoeopathy and the American Medical Association—Science and Ethics in American Medicine, 1800–1914*. 2d ed. Berkeley, Calif.: North Atlantic Books, 1982.

Dearborn, Earl H. "The Development of Pharmacology at Boston University School of Medicine." *Boston Medical Quarterly* 6, no. 2 (June 1955).

Deutsch, Sarah. "Learning to Talk More Like a Man: Boston Women's Class-Bridging Organization, 1870–1940." *American Historical Review* 97, no. 2 (April 1992).

Dinges, Martin, ed. *Patients in the History of Homoeopathy*. Sheffield, UK: European Association for the History of Medicine and Health Publications, 2002.

Drachman, Virginia G. "Gynecological Instruments and Surgical Decisions at a Hospital in Late-Nineteenth-Century America." *Journal of American Culture* 3 (1980).

———. "The Limits of Progress: The Professional Lives of Women Doctors, 1881–1926." In *Bulletin of the History of Medicine* 60 (spring 1986).

———. "Women Doctors and the Women's Medical Movement: Feminism and Medicine, 1850–1895." Ph.D. diss., State University of New York at Buffalo, 1976.

Duffy, Michael P. "A Progression of Sectarianism: Homeopathy in Massachusetts from 1855 to 1875." Bachelor's thesis, Harvard University, 1982.

Fee, Elizabeth, and Nancy Krieger, eds. *Women's Health, Politics, and Power: Essays on Sex/Gender, Medicine, and Public Health*. Amityville, N.Y.: Baywood Publishing Co., 1994.

Fox, Daniel M. *Health Policies and Health Politics: The British and American Experience, 1911–1965*. Princeton: Princeton University Press, 1986.

Freedman, Estelle. "Separatism as Strategy: Female Institution Building and American Feminism." *Feminist Studies* 53 (1979).

Fuller, Robert C. *Alternative Medicine and American Religious Life*. New York: Oxford University Press, 1989.

Gevitz, Norman, ed. *Other Healers: Unorthodox Medicine in America*. Baltimore: Johns Hopkins University Press, 1988

Glazer, Penina Migdal, and Miriam Slater. *Unequal Colleagues: The Entrance of Women into the Professions, 1890–1940*. New Brunswick, N.J.: Rutgers University Press, 1987.

Gordon, Linda. *Woman's Body, Woman's Right: Birth Control in America*. Rev. ed. New York: Penguin Books, 1990.

Haller, John S. Jr., and Barbara Mason. *Forging a Medical Practice, 1884–1938 An Illinois Case Study: Wilber Price Armstrong*. The Pearson Museum, Southern Illinois University, 1997.

Hine, Darlene Clark. "Co-Laborers in the Work of the Lord." In *The Racial Economy of Science: Toward a Democrtic Future*. Edited by Sandra Harding. Bloomington: Indiana University Press, 1993.

Hunt, Marion. "From Child Saving to Pediatrics: A Case Study of Women's Role in the Development of Saint Louis Children's Hospital, 1879–1925." Ph.D. diss., Washington University, 1992.

Jordanova, Ludmilla. *Sexual Visions: Images of Gender in Science and Medicine between the Eighteenth and Twentieth Centuries*. Madison: University of Wisconsin Press, 1989.

Jutte, Robert, Guenter B. Risse, and John Woodward. *Culture, Knowledge, and Healing: Historical Perspectives of Homeopathic Medicine in Europe and North America*. Sheffield, UK: European Association for the History of Medicine and Health Publications, 1998.

Kaufman, Martin. "The Admission of Women to Nineteenth-Century American Medical Societies." *Bulletin of the History of Medicine* 50 (1976).

———. *Homeopathy in America: The Rise and Fall of a Medical Heresy*. Baltimore: Johns Hopkins University Press, 1971.

Kett, Joseph F. *The Formation of the American Medical Profession: The Role of Institutions, 1780–1860*. New Haven: Yale University Press, 1968.

Kirschmann, Anne Taylor. "Struggle for Survival: The American Foundation for Homeopathy and the Preservation of Homoeopathy in the United States, 1920–1930." *Patients in the History of Homoeopathy*, Edited by Martin Dinges. Sheffield, UK: European Association for the History of Medicine and Health Publications, 2002.

———. "Adding Women to the Ranks, 1860–1890: A New View with a Homeopathic Lens." *Bulletin of the History of Medicine* 73 (fall 1999).

Lawrence, Christopher, and George Weisz, eds. *Greater than the Parts: Holism in Biomedicine, 1920–1950*. New York: Oxford University Press, 1998.

Lears, Jackson T. J. *No Place of Grace: Antimodernism and the Transformation of American Culture, 1880–1920*. Chicago: University of Chicago Press, 1981.

Leavitt, Judith Walzer, ed. *Women and Health in America: Historical Readings*. Madison: University of Wisconsin Press, 1984.

———, and Ronald L. Numbers, eds. *Sickness and Health in America: Readings in the History of Medicine and Public Health*. Madison: University of Wisconsin Press, 1985.

Linkugel, William A., and Martha Solomon. *Anna Howard Shaw: Suffrage Orator and Social Reformer*. Westport, Conn.: Greenwood Press, 1991.

Longo, Lawrence D. "The Rise and Fall of Battey's Operation: A Fashion in Surgery." *Bulletin of the History of Medicine* 53 (1979).

Lord, Alexandra. "'The Great *Arcana* of the Deity': Menstruation and Menstrual Disorders in Eighteenth-Century British Medical Thought." *Bulletin of the History of Medicine* 73 (spring 1999).

Ludmerer, Kenneth M. *Learning to Heal: The Development of American Medical Education*. New York: Basic Books, 1985.

Markowitz, Gerald E., and David Rosner. "Doctors in Crisis: Medical Education and Medical Reform During the Progressive Era, 1895–1915." In *Health Care in America: Essays in Social History*. Edited by Susan Reverby and David Rosner. Philadelphia: Temple University Press, 1979.

Marks, Harry M. *The Progress of Experiment: Science and Therapeutic Reform in the United States, 1900–1990*. Cambridge: Cambridge University Press, 1997.

Marrett, Cora Bagley. "On the Evolution of Women's Medical Societies." In *Women and Health in America*. Edited by Judith Walzer Leavitt. Madison: University of Wisconsin Press, 1984.

———. "Influences on the Rise of New Organizations: The Formation of Women's Medical Societies." *Administrative Science Quarterly* 25 (June 1980).

Moldow, Gloria. *Women Doctors in Gilded-Age Washington: Race, Gender, and Profes-sionalization.* Urbana and Chicago: University of Illinois Press, 1987.

Morantz-Sanchez, Regina Markell. *Sympathy and Science: Women Physicians in Ameri-can Medicine.* New York: Oxford University Press, 1985.

———. "Entering Male Professional Terrain: Dr. Mary Dixon Jones and the Emer-gence of Gynecological Surgery in the Nineteenth-Century United States." *Gen-der and History* 7, no. 2 (August 1995).

———. "Feminist Theory and Historical Practice: Rereading Elizabeth Blackwell." *History and Theory: Studies in the Philosophy of History* Beiheft 31 (December 1992).

———. "Making Women Modern: Middle-Class Women and Health Reform in America." In *Women and Health in America.* Edited by Judith Walzer Leavitt. Madison: University of Wisconsin Press, 1984.

———. "The 'Connecting Link': The Case for the Woman Doctor in Nineteenth Century America." In *Sickness and Health in America: Readings in the History of Medicine and Public Health,* 2d ed. Edited by Judith Walzer Leavitt and Ronald L. Numbers. Madison: University of Wisconsin Press, 1985.

———. "The Perils of Feminist History." In *Women and Health in America.* Edited by Judith Walzer Leavitt. Madison: University of Wisconsin Press, 1984.

More, Ellen S. *Restoring the Balance: Women Physicians and the Profession of Medicine, 1850–1995.* Cambridge and London: Harvard University Press, 1999.

———. "The American Medical Women's Association and the Role of the Woman Physician, 1915–1990." *Journal of the American Medical Women's Association* 45, no. 5 (September/October 1990).

———. "The Blackwell Medical Society and the Professionalization of Women Physi-cians." *Bulletin of the History of Medicine* 61 (1987).

Moscucci, Ornella. *The Science of Woman: Gynaecology and Gender in England 1800–1929.* Cambridge: Cambridge University Press, 1990.

Myerson, Joel, Daniel Shealy, and Madeleine B. Stern, eds. *The Selected Letters of Louisa May Alcott.* Boston and Toronto: Little, Brown & Co., 1987.

Newman, Charlotte S. "Cleveland's First Woman Physician: Myra Merrick Struggled to Bring Medical Care to the Poor." *The Gamut* 216 (spring 1989).

Nicholls, Phillip A. *Homeopathy and the Medical Profession.* London: Croom Helm, 1988.

Numbers, Ronald L. "Do-It-Yourself the Sectarian Way" in *"Send Us a Lady Physician" Women Doctors in America, 1835–1920.* Edited by Ruth J. Abram. New York: W. W. Norton & Co., 1985.

———. "The Fall and Rise of the American Medical Profession," in *Sickness and Health in America: Readings in the History of Medicine and Public Health.* Edited by Judith Walzer Leavitt and Ronald L. Numbers. Madison: University of Wisconsin Press, 1985.

Parker, Gail, ed. *The Oven Birds: American Women on Womanhood, 1820–1920.* Gar-den City, N.Y.: Anchor Books, 1972.

Parsons, Gail Pat. "Equal Treatment for All: American Medical Remedies for Male Sexual Problems, 1850–1900." *Journal of the History of Medicine and Allied Sciences* 31, no. 1 (January 1977).

Peck, Phoebe. "Women Physicians and their State Medical Societies." *Journal of the American Medical Women's Association* 20, no. 4 (April 1965).

Pernick, Martin. *A Calculus of Suffering: Pain, Professionalism, and Anesthesia in Nine-teenth Century America.* New York: Columbia University Press, 1985.

Porter, Roy. *The Greatest Benefit to Mankind: A Medical History of Humanity.* New York: W. W. Norton & Co., 1997.

Ricci, James V. *The Development of Gynaecological Surgery and Instruments: A Compre-*

hensive Review of the Evolution of Surgery and Surgical Instruments for the Treatment of Female Diseases from the Hippocratic Age to the Antiseptic Period. Philadelphia and Toronto: Blakiston Co., 1949.

Roberts, William H. "Orthodoxy vs. Homeopathy: Ironic Developments Following the Flexner Report at the Ohio State University." *Bulletin of the History of Medicine* 60 (1986).

Rogers, Naomi. "The Public Face of Homoeopathy: Politics, the Public, and Alternative Medicine in the United States, 1900–1940." In *Patients in the History of Homoeopathy*. Edited by Martin Dinges. Sheffield, UK: European Association for the History of Medicine and Health Publications, 1998.

———. "American Homeopathy Confronts Scientific Medicine." In *Culture, Knowledge, and Healing: Historical Perspectives of Homeopathic Medicine in Europe and North America*. Edited by Robert, Jutte, Guenter B. Risse, and John Woodward. Sheffield, UK: European Association for the History of Medicine and Health Publications, 1998.

———. "The Proper Place of Homeopathy: Hahnemann Medical College and Hospital in an Age of Scientific Medicine." *Pennsylvania Magazine of History and Biography* 108 (1984).

———. "Women and Sectarian Medicine." In *Women, Health, and Medicine in America: A Historical Handbook*. Edited by Rima D. Apple. New Brunswick, N.J.: Rutgers University Press, 1992.

———. *An Alternative Path: The Making and Remaking of Hahnemann Medical College and Hospital of Philadelphia*. New Brunswick, N.J.: Rutgers University Press, 1998.

Rosenberg, Charles E. "Holism in Twentieth-Century Medicine." In *Greater than the Parts: Holism in Biomedicine, 1920–1950*. Edited by Christopher Lawrence and George Weisz. New York: Oxford University Press, 1998.

———. "Introduction: Science, Society, and Social Thought." In *No Other Gods: On Science and American Social Thought*. Baltimore: Johns Hopkins University Press, 1976.

———. "The Therapeutic Revolution: Medicine, Meaning, and Social Change in Nineteenth-Century America." In *Perspectives in Biology and Medicine* 20 (1977).

———, ed. *The Origins of Specialization in American Medicine: An Anthology of Sources*. New York and London: Garland Publishing, 1989.

———. "The Therapeutic Revolution: Medicine, Meaning, and Social Change in Nineteenth-Century America." In *The Therapeutic Revolution: Essays on the Social History of American Medicine*. Edited by Morris Vogel and Charles E. Rosenberg. Philadelphia: University of Pennsylvania Press, 1979.

Rosenkrantz, Barbara Gutmann. "The Search for Professional Order in Nineteenth Century American Medicine." In *Sickness & Health in America: Readings in the History of Medicine and Public Health*. Edited by Judith Walzer Leavitt and Ronald L. Numbers. Madison: University of Wisconsin Press, 1985.

Rosner, David. *A Once Charitable Enterprise*. Princeton: Princeton University Press, 1987.

Rothstein, William G. *American Medical Schools and the Practice of Medicine*. New York: Oxford University Press, 1987.

———. *American Physicians in the Nineteenth Century: From Sects to Science*. Baltimore: Johns Hopkins University Press, 1985.

Roy, Judith M. "Surgical Gynecology." In *Women, Health, and Medicine in America: A Historical Handbook*. Edited by Rima D. Apple. New Brunswick, N.J.: Rutgers University Press, 1990.

Schiebinger, Londa. *The Mind Has No Sex? Women in the Origins of Modern Science*. Cambridge: Harvard University Press, 1989.

Schmidt, Josef M. "Homeopathy in the American West: Its German Connections." In *Culture, Knowledge, and Healing: Historical Perspectives of Homeopathic Medicine in Europe and North America*. Edited by Robert Jutte, Guenter B. Risse and John Woodward. Sheffield, UK: European Association for the History of Medicine and Health Publications, 1998.

Selmon, Bertha L. "Early Development of Medical Opportunity for Women in the United States, 1850–1879." *Medical Woman's Journal* (January 1947).

———. "The New York Medical College and Hospital for Women." *Medical Woman's Journal* (April 1946).

Seraile, William. "Susan McKinney Steward: New York State's First African-American Woman Physician." *Afro-Americans in New York Life and History* 9, no. 2 (1985).

Shifrin, Susan. "From the kingdom of fancy, fashion and foolery, to the kingdom of reason and righteousness . . . : Dress Reform and the Constraints of Clothing on Women Physicians at the Woman's Medical College of Pennsylvania, 1850–1900." In *Collections: The Newsletter of the Archives and Special Collections on Women in Medicine* 27 (October 1993).

Shorter, Edward. *From Paralysis to Fatigue: A History of Psychosomatic Illness in the Modern Era*. New York: The Free Press, 1992.

———. *The History of Women's Bodies*. New York: Basic Books, 1982.

———. *Women's Bodies: A Social History of Women's Encounter with Health, Ill-Health, and Medicine*. New Brunswick, N.J.: Transaction Publishers, 1991.

Shortt, S.E.D. "Physicians, Science, and Status: Issues in the Professionalization of Anglo-American Medicine in the Nineteenth Century." *Medical History* 27 (1983).

Shryock, Richard H. "Empiricism versus Rationalism in American Medicine, 1650–1950." *Proceedings of the American Antiquarian Society* 79 (1969).

Smith-Rosenberg, Carroll, and Charles E. Rosenberg. "The Female Animal: Medical and Biological Views of Woman and Her Role in Nineteenth Century America." In *Women and Health in America: Historical Readings*. Edited by Judith Walzer Leavitt. Madison: University of Wisconsin Press, 1984.

Solberg, Winton U. "Martha G. Ripley: Pioneer Doctor and Social Reformer." *Minnesota History* 39, no. 1 (spring 1964).

Stansell, Christine. "Elizabeth Stuart Phelps: A Study in Female Rebellion." *Massachusetts Review* 13 (1979).

Starr, Paul. *The Social Transformation of American Medicine*. New York: Basic Books, 1982.

Staudt, Dorte. "The Roles of Laymen in the History of German Homeopathy." In *Culture, Knowledge, and Healing: Historical Perspectives of Homeopathic Medicine in Europe and North America*. Edited by Robert Jutte, Guenter B. Risse, and John Woodward. Sheffield, UK: European Association for the History of Medicine and Health Publications, 1998.

Sterling, Dorothy, ed. *We Are Your Sisters: Black Women in the Nineteenth Century*. New York: W. W. Norton, 1984.

Stevens, Rosemary. "The Changing Idea of a Medical Specialty." *Transactions and Studies of the College of Physicians of Philadelphia* 5 (1980).

———. *In Sickness and in Wealth: American Hospitals in the Twentieth Century*. New York: Basic Books, 1989.

Stowe, Steven. "Seeing Themselves at Work: Physicians and the Case Narrative in the Mid-Nineteenth-Century American South." *American Historical Review* 101, no. 1 (February 1996).

Theriot, Nancy M. "Women's Voices in the Nineteenth-Century Medical Discourse: A Step Toward Deconstructing Science." *Signs* 29 (1993).

Verbrugge, Martha. *Able-Bodied Womanhood: Personal Health and Social Change in Nineteenth-Century Boston*. New York: Oxford University Press, 1988.

Vogel, Morris. *The Invention of the Modern Hospital: Boston, 1870–1930*. Chicago: Chicago University Press, 1980.

Walsh, Mary Roth. *"Doctors Wanted: No Women Need Apply" Sexual Barriers in the Medical Profession, 1835–1975*. New Haven: Yale University Press, 1977.

Warner, John Harley. "Remembering Paris: Memory and the American Disciples of French Medicine in the Nineteenth Century." *Bulletin of the History of Medicine* 65 (1991).

———. "Science in Medicine." *OSIRIS* 2, no. 1 (1985).

———. "The Fall and Rise of Professional Mystery: Epistemology, Authority, and the Emergence of Laboratory Medicine in Nineteenth-Century America." In *The Laboratory Revolution in Medicine*. Edited by Andrew Cunningham and Perry Williams. Cambridge: Cambridge University Press, 1992.

———. *Against the Spirit of System: The French Impulse in Nineteenth-Century American Medicine*. Princeton: Princeton University Press, 1998.

———. *The Therapeutic Perspective: Medical Practice, Knowledge, and Identity in America, 1820–1885*. Cambridge: Harvard University Press, 1986.

———. "Medical Sectarianism, Therapeutic Conflict, and the Shaping of Orthodox Professional Identity in Antebellum American Medicine." In *Medical Fringe and Medical Orthodoxy, 1750–1850*. Edited by W. F. Bynum and Roy Porter. London: Croom Helm, 1987.

———. "Orthodoxy and Otherness: Homeopathy and Regular Medicine in Nineteenth-Century America." In *Culture, Knowledge, and Healing: Historical Perspectives of Homeopathic Medicine in Europe and North America*. Edited by Robert Jutte, Guenter B. Risse, and John Woodward. Sheffield, UK: European Association for the History of Medicine and Health Publications, 1998.

Wershub, Leonard Paul. *One Hundred Years of Medical Progress: A History of the New York Medical College Flower and Fifth Avenue Hospitals*. Springfield, Ill.: Charles C. Thomas, 1967.

Winston, Julian. "A Modern Biography of James Tyler Kent." *The American Homeopath* 2 (1995).

———. *The Faces of Homoeopathy: An Illustrated History of the First 200 Years*. Tawa, NZ: Great Awk Publishing, 1999.

Wittern, Renate. "The Origins of Homoeopathy in Germany." *Clio Medica* 22 (1991).

Wood, Ann Douglas. "'The Fashionable Diseases': Women's Complaints and their Treatment in Nineteenth-Century America." In *Women and Health in America*. Edited by Judith Walzer Leavitt. Madison: University of Wisconsin Press, 1984.

Index

About the Author

Anne Taylor Kirschmann received her Ph.D. in American history at the University of Rochester in 1999. A historian of medicine, she has published on the history of alternative medicine and women in medicine. She is currently a lecturer in history at the University of Massachusetts, Dartmouth, and is re-examining the role of social reformer Mary Ware Dennett in the early-twentieth-century birth control and sex education movement.